POCKET BOOK ON
TRAY AND TROLLEY SETTING

THE AUTHOR

Helen M. Dickie
R.G.N., R.F.N., S.C.M.
Sister Tutor, Peliminary Training School
Southern General Hospital, Glasgow

FOREWORD BY

I. G. McInroy
M.B.E., R.G.N., S.C.M., D.N.(London)
Formerly Principal Sister Tutor, Glasgow Royal Infirmary
Formerly Member of the General Nursing Council for Scotland

POCKET BOOK ON
TRAY AND TROLLEY SETTING

Helen M. Dickie

Foreword by
I. G. McInroy

FIFTH EDITION

E. & S. LIVINGSTONE
EDINBURGH AND LONDON
1970

First Edition	.	. 1959
Second Edition	.	. 1961
Third Edition	.	. 1963
Fourth Edition	.	. 1966
Reprinted .	.	. 1968
Fifth Edition	.	. 1970

I.S.B.N. 0 443 00706 3

Made and Printed in Great Britain

FOREWORD

At the present time an increasing amount of professional knowledge is demanded from the student nurse and it is not difficult to understand why the task of memorising details of practical ward procedures becomes a burden to her. This applies particularly to the junior nurse, who is often bewildered by the number of new subjects she requires to learn during her first year. Miss Dickie, as the result of her teaching experience in the Preliminary Training School for Student Nurses in a large general hospital, is well aware of this problem.

Not every hospital ward possesses a procedure book, and this pocket handbook provides information on tray and trolley setting in a concise form. It contains lists of requirements for the majority of ward treatments and clear line drawings to help those who are visually perceptive. Standardisation is almost impossible and only minor differences in method exist between one hospital and another.

A chapter on methods of sterilisation is an added asset as the problem of cross infection in hospital wards is giving concern to both the medical and nursing professions.

The newly qualified nurse and ward sister will welcome this book as an aid to ward teaching, and it should find a place in the classroom and on the ward desk. Miss Dickie has given much time and thought to the preparation of this book, and it will, I am sure, prove itself to be a useful and popular reference book.

I. G. McINROY.

1959.

PREFACE TO THE FIFTH EDITION

ANY alteration in the content of this edition has been influenced by the ever-increasing range of disposable equipment now available and the introduction of the metric system.

A decade has elapsed since the first edition was published. Considerable change in the content and scope of nurse-training has evolved during this period. There would appear, however, to be a continuing demand for a pocket book of this kind.

My sincere thanks to the many nurses, from the hospital service and elsewhere, who have indicated that the book has proved useful to them in their particular branch of nursing.

H. M. DICKIE.

1970.

PREFACE TO FIRST EDITION

THERE is an old Chinese proverb which states: "A thousand hearings are not as good as one seeing." The subject of visual aids in teaching is receiving considerable attention to-day. No one concerned with nurse training can afford to overlook the opportunities in this field.

In compiling this little book no attempt has been made to include every tray and trolley which the nurse may require to prepare in her routine ward work. However, using the General Nursing Council (Scotland) Syllabus as a guide, I have endeavoured to include illustrations for most practical procedures carried out at the bedside.

We do well to remember the words of the International Code of Nursing Ethics—" Service to mankind is the primary function of nurses and the reason for the existence of the nursing profession." I trust therefore that the use of the book may not only help nurses in training to overcome some difficulties, but may result in some valuable time being saved in these days when the cry echoes through so many of our hospital wards, " No time to nurse." The pages which have been left throughout for notes will, I hope, serve a useful purpose.

With the existent diversity of thought on nursing procedures standardisation is not easily accomplished, but that it could be is not in doubt. In view of this diversity it has been no easy task to try to reach a point midway between oversimplification and undue elaboration, but this has been aimed at in the preparation of illustrations.

No doubt all are familiar with the fact that syringes can be sterilised by autoclaving, exposure in the hot air oven, the use of infra-red radiation or, if they are of the disposable variety, discarded after use. The administration of an enema saponis, to mention only one extremely familiar procedure, can now be carried out with the minimum of effort, time and equipment. As such advances continue, the requirements for practical procedures must of necessity change, but whatever the change in pattern may be the basic nursing needs of the patient will emerge unaltered. More advanced techniques will certainly be joined by others equally complex and requiring the intelligent co-operation of the nurse at every stage.

The fact that we are on the eve of exciting developments in the sphere of nursing in this country cannot be disputed. The rumblings of the past two decades from within the profession are gaining in momentum from those arising as a result of external pressures. In the midst of this scene of change the earnest desire of all engaged in this service to humanity is that an atmosphere may be created conducive to the patient's physical, social and spiritual well-being.

H. M. DICKIE.

Glasgow, 1959.

ACKNOWLEDGMENTS

WITHOUT the helpful suggestions and criticisms received from many of my colleagues this book could never have been completed. In thanking all who helped and encouraged, I would specially mention Miss I. G. McInroy, Principal Tutor, Royal Infirmary, Glasgow, for valuable suggestions made and kindly consenting to write the Foreword; and Mr R. H. G. Christie, Principal Tutor, Preliminary Training School, Southern General Hospital, Glasgow, who gave so willingly of his time in consideration of requirements necessary for each procedure and in checking of the proofs. I would extend my sincere thanks to Mr Charles Macmillan for help and encouragement given, Mr James Parker and all other members of the staff of E. & S. Livingstone who have helped in the preparation and publication of this book.

I would acknowledge a great debt and express my thanks to the artist, Mr R. Callander, for the excellent way in which he prepared all illustrations.

H. M. DICKIE.

ACKNOWLEDGMENTS

H. McDIESH.

POCKET BOOK ON
TRAY AND TROLLEY SETTING

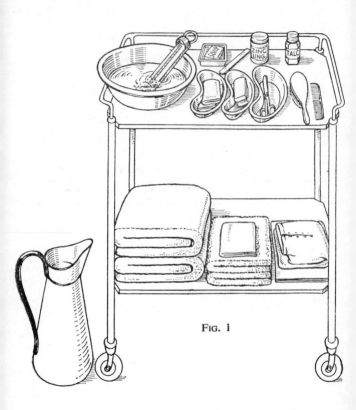

FIG. 1

2

Fig. 1

Trolley for bathing a patient in bed

1. A large basin of water at the correct temperature, 105° F. (40·5° C.).
2. A bath thermometer.
3. Soap in a soap dish.
4. Two face cloths in a receiver.
5. A nail brush in a receiver.
6. Scissors in a large receiver.
7. A hair brush and comb.
8. A jar of talcum powder.
9. A jar of zinc and castor oil ointment and a wooden spatula (or other suitable application for pressure areas).

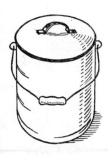

10. Two bathing sheets (preferably of terry towelling or flannelette, and changed for each patient).
11. Two bath towels.
12. A face towel.
13. A jug with fresh water.
14. Clean nightdress and bed linen as required.
15. A bucket for soiled water.

(Protect the bed and the floor as required.)

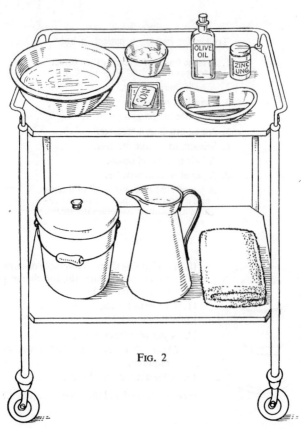

Fig. 2

FIG. 2

Trolley for routine local treatment of the pressure areas

1. A basin of warm water.
2. Soap in a soap dish.
3. A bowl with cotton-wool mops.
4. A receiver or disposal bag for discarded material.
5. A suitable application for the pressure areas, *e.g.*, zinc and castor oil ointment (and wooden spatula).
   Olive oil.
   A barrier cream.
   Silicone spray.

6. Patient's own treatment towel to dry the part.
7. A large jug of fresh water.
8. A bucket for soiled water.

N.B.—Local application to the pressure areas must be supplementary to:
        Frequent change of position when possible.
        Adequate nutrition of the patient.
        Attention to general cleanliness.

Use of measures to relieve pressure, *e.g.*
        Water beds.
        Plastic foam mattresses.
        Alternating air pressure mattresses.
        Tubipad.
        Sheepskin.
        Foam heel rest.

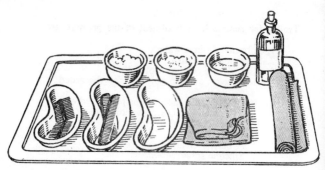

FIG. 3

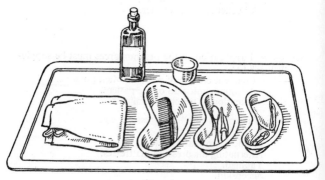

FIG. 4

Fig. 3

Tray for routine inspection of the hair

1. A bottle of suitable antiseptic solution.
2. A small bowl.
3. Fine tooth combs in a receiver.
4. Dressing combs in a receiver.
5. A bowl with white cotton-wool mops.
6. A bowl with brown wool mops.
7. A receiver or disposal bag for soiled wool
   mops.
8. A plastic shoulder cape.
9. Polythene to protect bed as required.

Fig. 4

Tray for treatment of a verminous head

1. A bottle of lorexane.
2. A gallipot.
3. A dressing comb in a receiver.
4. An old teaspoon or a pipette in a receiver.
5. A triangular bandage and a safety-pin or
   disposable cap.
6. A plastic shoulder cape.

(Nurse protects herself by wearing a gown
and disposable cap.)

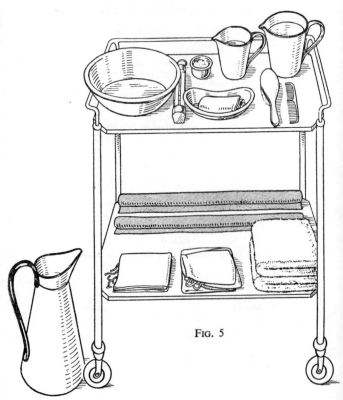

F<small>IG</small>. 5

8

FIG. 5

Trolley for washing a patient's hair in bed

1. A large basin.
2. A bath thermometer.
3. A small bowl with cotton-wool mops (for ears if desired).
4. A face cloth in a receiver.
5. A small jug of shampoo.
6. A large jug for rinsing water.
7. A hair brush and comb.

8. A waterproof pillowslip.
9. A plastic cape.
10. Two bath towels.
11. Polythene sheeting to protect bed and floor as required.
12. A large jug with the supply of rinsing water.
13. A bucket for soiled water.

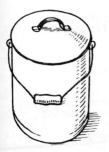

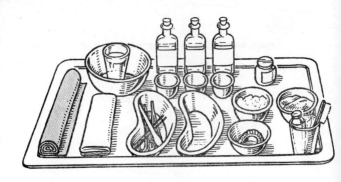

Fig. 6

Tray for cleaning the mouth

1. A polythene square.
2. A disposable drape.
3. A mouth wash in a tumbler or feeding cup (glycothymoline, 1 : 10).
4. A bowl for the return wash.
5. Three bottles of lotion : soda bicarbonate solution; glycothymoline, 1 : 10; glycerine of borax.
6. Three gallipots.
7. Cold cream for the lips.
8. A bowl with white cotton-wool mops.
9. A bowl with gauze swabs.
10. A bowl for the dentures.
11. A receiver or disposal bag for soiled swabs.
12. A large receiver with artery forceps, dissecting forceps, wooden probes and spatula.
13. The patient's own tooth brush and paste.

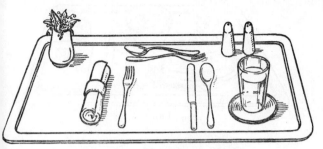

FIG. 7

Lunch tray for convalescent patient

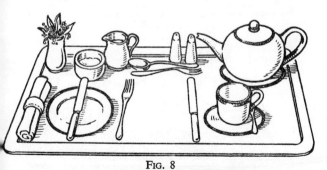

FIG. 8

Breakfast tray for convalescent patient

11

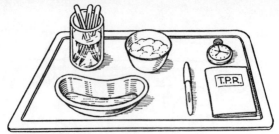

Fig. 9

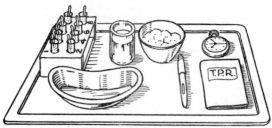

Fig. 10

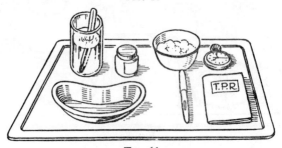

Fig. 11

FIG. 9

Trays for taking body temperature

In the axilla or groin—

1. Thermometers in an uncovered jar containing disinfectant, the bulbs resting on a pad of cotton-wool.
2. A bowl with cotton-wool mops.
3. A receiver for soiled mops.
4. A watch with a seconds hand.
5. A fountain pen.
6. A book or a chart on which to record findings.

FIG. 10

In the mouth—

1. Individual thermometers in jars as before, but these may be in a labelled stand or fixed to the wall behind the patient's bed.
2. A bowl with cotton-wool mops.
3. A receiver for soiled mops.
4. A watch with a seconds hand.
5. A jar with water in which to rinse the thermometer on removal from the disinfectant.
6. A fountain pen.
7. A book or chart on which to record findings.

FIG. 11

In the rectum—

1. A special rectal thermometer with a coloured bulb, in a jar as before.
2. A bowl with cotton-wool mops.
3. A receiver for soiled mops.
4. A jar with petroleum jelly to lubricate the thermometer before it is inserted.
5. A watch with a seconds hand.
6. A fountain pen.
7. A book or chart on which to record findings.

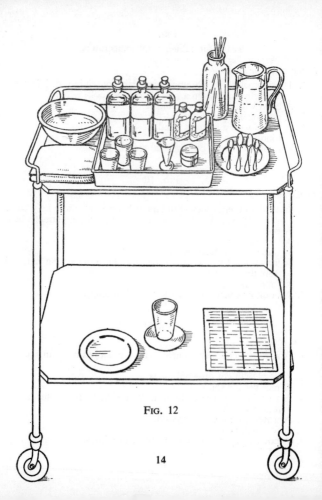

Fig. 12

Fig. 12
Basic trolley for administration of medicines orally

1. A tray with the following :
   - Bottles of mixtures.
   - Pills and tablets.
   - Powders and cachets, etc.
   - Medicine glasses graduated in millilitres.
2. A jug of cold water.
3. A jar with drinking straws and a glass stirring rod.
4. A plate with various sizes of spoons
5. A basin of warm water.
6. A medicine towel.

7. Individual treatment cards.
8. A tumbler and a saucer.
9. A plate on which to place the spoon or medicine glass.

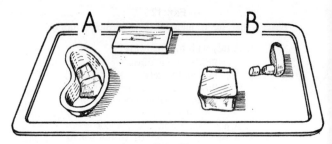

Fig. 13

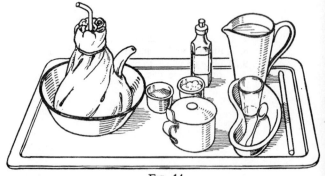

Fig. 14

Fig. 13

Tray for a dry inhalation

A. Without inhaler, *e.g.*,
    1. Amyl nitrite capsule.
    2. Gauze swab in which to crush capsule.
    Vapour inhaled cautiously for relief of angina pectoris.

B. With an inhaler, *e.g.*,
    1. Medihaler.
    2. Pressurised vial containing drug such as isoprenaline sulphate.
    Application of pressure on vial delivers a measured dose of the drug.

N.B.—One to two inhalations only at a time for relief of broncho-spasm.

Fig. 14

Tray for a moist inhalation

1. An earthenware inhaler.
2. A flannel bag to cover the inhaler (spout always exposed).
3. A bowl in which to stand the inhaler.
4. A gallipot with a gauze swab to wrap round the mouthpiece.
5. A bottle with the drug, *e.g.*, tincture of benzoin compound.
6. A gallipot with a wool mop on which to place the drug.
7. A receiver with a teaspoon or graduated measure.
8. A jug with 600 ml. of water at 160° F. (71·1° C.).
9. A lotion thermometer.
10. A disposable sputum carton.

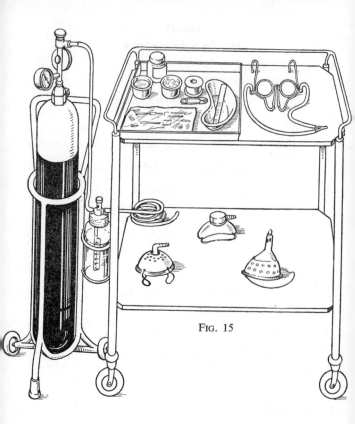

FIG. 15

Fig. 15
Requirements for administration of oxygen

1. A cylinder of oxygen with pressure gauge, fine adjustment valve, stand and cylinder key; *or* a " pipe line " supply to the bedside.
2. Combined flowmeter and humidifier.

3. Rubber tubing from cylinder to humidifier.
4. Rubber tubing and a connection from humidifier to the apparatus being used for administering, *e.g.*,

   (*a*) Nasal catheter. Tray as follows :

   > Packet with sterile disposable nasal catheters.
   > Gallipot with cotton-wool mops.
   > Gallipot with warm saline solution.
   > A lubricant, *e.g.*, petroleum jelly or cocaine ointment and a wooden spatula.
   > Adhesive strapping and a safety-pin.
   > Receiver for soiled cotton-wool.

   (Tudor Edwards' spectacle frame may be substituted for nasal catheters on tray.)

   (*b*) Disposable Oronasal Mask, *e.g.*,

   > Ventimask (rate 4-6 litres per minute). This gives a low concentration of oxygen, *e.g.*, 28 per cent. and is used when controlled oxygen therapy is essential as in chronic bronchitis.
   > The Edinburgh mask is similar in principle to Ventimask and also gives low concentration of oxygen.
   > MC (Mac) mask (rate 6 to 8 litres per minute). This gives a higher concentration of oxygen, *e.g.*, 40 to 60 per cent.

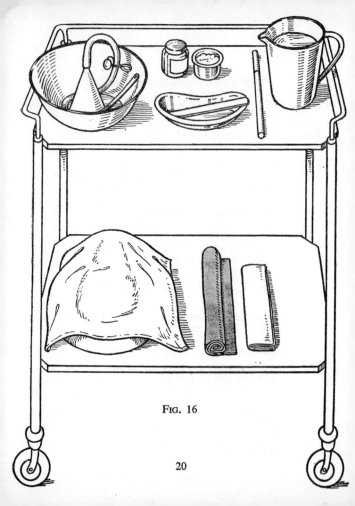

Fig. 16

20

FIG. 16
Trolley for an evacuant enema

1. A large bowl with the apparatus, *i.e.*, a catheter (No. 12), connection, tubing, funnel and clamp.
2. A jar of petroleum jelly and wooden spatula.
3. A gallipot with cotton-wool mops.
4. A receiver or disposal bag for soiled mops.
5. A jug with the enema soap solution at the correct temperature, 100° F. (37·7° C.).
6. Lotion thermometer.

7. Polythene to protect bed.
8. A disposable drape.
9. A heated bed pan and cover.

Alternatively.—A disposable enema unit may be used when available. (See overleaf for apparatus.)

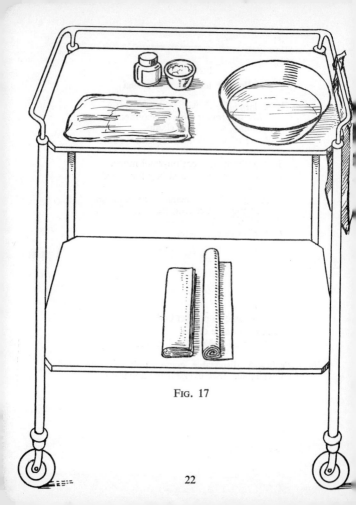

FIG. 17

FIG. 17

Tray or trolley for a retention enema

1. Bowl with warm water in which to heat the unit.
2. A lubricant such as petroleum jelly; a wooden spatula.
3. A gallipot with cotton-wool mops.
4. A disposable enema unit, *e.g.*,

   (*a*) 130 ml. oil (arachis or olive oil) may be used to soften impacted or hard fæces.
   (*b*) 130 ml. magnesium sulphate solution may be used as an adjunct to neurosurgery.
   (*c*) Solution of cortisone may be used in the treatment of ulcerative colitis.

5. Disposal bag.

6. Polythene to protect bed.
7. Disposable drape.

A bed elevator may be required in order to aid retention of the solution.

(The disposable unit used for an evacuant enema contains 120 ml. of a solution of phosphates.)

2   23

NOTES

NOTES

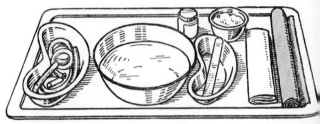

FIG. 18

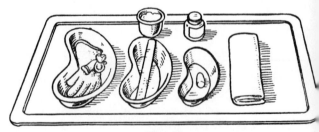

FIG. 19

Fig. 18

Tray for passing a flatus tube

1. A large receiver with the flatus tube and extra rubber tubing and connection when required.
2. A bowl of warm water to which an antiseptic has been added.
3. A jar of petroleum jelly and wooden spatula.
4. A gallipot with cotton-wool mops.
5. A receiver or disposal bag for soiled mops.
6. Polythene.
7. Disposable drape.

Fig. 19

Tray for the administration of a suppository

1. A receiver with a finger cot or a rubber glove and a little bag of powder.
2. A small receiver with the suppository.
3. A gallipot with cotton-wool mops.
4. A jar of petroleum jelly and wooden spatula.
5. A receiver or disposal bag for soiled mops and gloves.
6. A disposable drape.

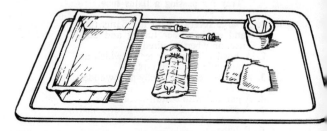

FIG. 20

Tray for hypodermic injection

1. Packet with sterile syringe.
2. Sterile hypodermic needles.
3. Small sterile disposable tray on which to take the charged syringe to the bedside.
4. The ordered drug, which may be in a " snap " ampoule or a rubber-capped bottle.
5. An ampoule file as required.
6. Sterile swabs impregnated with a skin disinfectant.

(Check written prescription before administration.)

NOTES

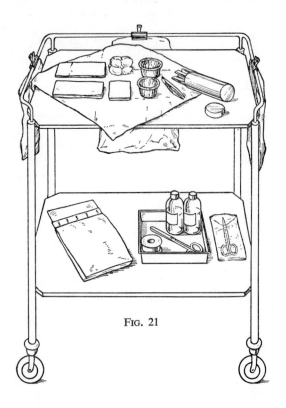

FIG. 21

Fig. 21
Trolley for a simple ward dressing

1. Contents of sterile dressings pack carefully removed from outer packet and left on opened out inner wrapping :

    One large disposable clinical sheet.
    Two cellulose squares.
    8 to 10 cotton-wool balls.
    4 to 6 gauze swabs.
    Two disposable gallipots.

    (Contents of pack will vary with dressing to be done.)

2. The required instruments are emptied out of metal container on to the sterile surface, *e.g.*, 3 to 4 pairs of dissecting forceps.

On lower shelf.

3. An unopened sterile dressings pack.
4. A small tray with the following :

    Bottles containing the required lotions, *e.g.*, eusol and a solution of hibitane and cetavlon.
    Adhesive plaster and a pair of dressings scissors.

5. One pair of sterile stitch scissors in a nylon film packet (the points of these are always protected with a piece of rubber tubing or a fold of foil).

N.B.—Dressings pack, instrument container and scissors packet should all be stamped with the date of sterilisation.

Three disposable bags are attached to the trolley with clips :

    One for soiled instruments.
    One for soiled dressings.
    A larger one at the back for the left-overs from each dressings pack.

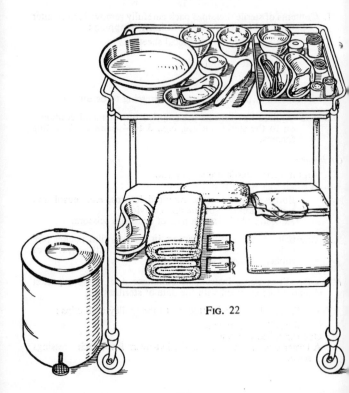

Fig. 22

32

FIG. 22

Trolley for the last offices

1. A basin of warm water to which a disinfectant has been added.
2. Soap in a soap dish.
3. A receiver with two washing flannels.
4. A bowl with white cotton-wool.
5. A bowl with brown wool.
6. A hair brush and comb.
7. A tray with sinus forceps, dressing forceps and scissors in a receiver. (If there is a dressing: a bowl of disinfectant and a receiver with dressings—elastoplast or adhesive.) Calico bandages and a roll of tape.

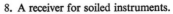

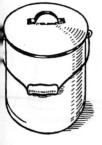

8. A receiver for soiled instruments.
9. Two bath towels.
10. Two correctly filled in mortuary cards with tapes.
11. A shroud.
12. A large pad of cotton-wool or gamgee.
13. A mortuary sheet (with some form of distinctive marking).
14. A bin or disposal bag for soiled dressings.
15. A receptacle for soiled linen.

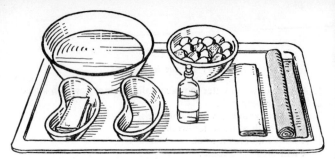

FIG. 23

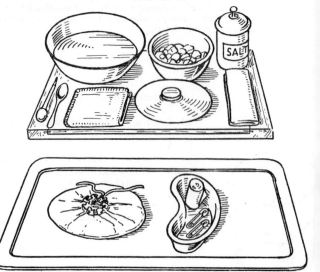

FIG. 24

34

Fig. 23

Tray for application of a cold compress

1. A bowl of cold water.
2. A bowl with pieces of ice.
3. Several single layers of old linen or lint in a receiver.
4. A receiver in which to place the compress on removal.
5. A treatment towel and mackintosh or jaconet.
6. A bottle of, *e.g.*, eau-de-Cologne or lavender water if being applied for the relief of headache.

(A bed cradle may be necessary if being applied over a joint.)

Fig. 24

An ice bag

To prepare—
1. A poultice board.
2. A bowl with chopped ice.
3. A bowl with tepid water (in which to swill the sharp edges off the ice).
4. A jar with salt.
5. A teaspoon.
6. An ice-pick.
7. A flannel square.
8. An ice bag.
9. A towel to dry the bag with.

To apply—Tray with :
1. The ice bag in a cover.
2. A receiver with a bandage and safety-pins.

(A bed cradle may be required from which to suspend the bag.)

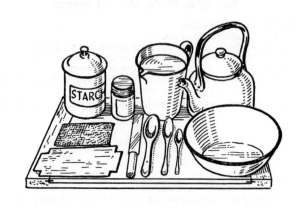

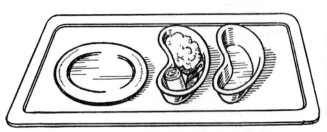

Fig. 25

FIG. 25

A starch poultice

To prepare—

1. A poultice board.
2. A jar with starch.
3. A jar with boracic powder.
4. A jug with cold water.
5. A kettle with boiling water.
6. A large bowl.
7. A teaspoon, a tablespoon and a wooden spoon.
8. A spatula
9. A piece of old linen cut and cornered.
10. A layer of gauze.

*To apply—*A tray with :

1. The poultice (cold) on a plate.
2. A receiver with a piece of cotton-wool, a bandage and a safety-pin.
3. A receiver for discarded poultice when necessary.

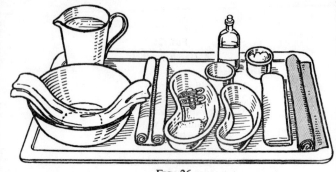

FIG. 26

Tray for a medical fomentation

1. A large bowl with the fomentation flannel folded inside a wringer.
2. A jug of boiling water.
3. A receiver with a square of jaconet (1 in. larger all round than the flannel), a square of cotton-wool (1 in. larger than the jaconet) and safety-pins.
4. A binder or bandage.
5. A treatment mackintosh and towel.

Whenever the skin appears to be tender:
    A bottle of olive oil and a gallipot.
    A gallipot with cotton-wool mops.
    A receiver for soiled mops.

When a surgical fomentation is required: as for Figure 21 with the addition of sterile, moist boracic lint.

NOTES

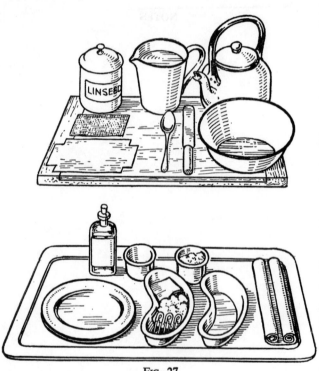

FIG. 27

Fig. 27

A linseed poultice

To prepare—

1. A poultice board.
2. A jar with linseed meal.
3. An enamel jug.
4. A kettle with boiling water.
5. A large enamel bowl.
6. A spatula.
7. A tablespoon.
8. A piece of old linen cut and cornered.
9. A single layer of gauze.

For a linseed and mustard poultice add to these requirements a jar of mustard.

*To apply—*A tray with the following :

1. Two well-heated plates (between which to place the poultice).
2. A receiver with a suitable-sized piece of jaconet and cotton-wool to cover the poultice, and several safety-pins.
3. A bottle of olive oil.
4. A gallipot for olive oil.
5. A gallipot with cotton-wool mops.
6. A receiver for soiled cotton-wool.
7. A bandage or binder.

For a linseed and mustard poultice requirements are similar, but omit the jaconet for covering the poultice.

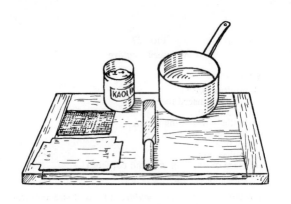

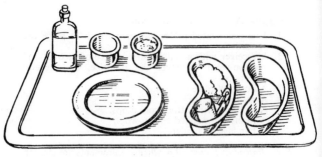

FIG. 28

Fig. 28

A kaolin poultice

To prepare—

1. A poultice board.
2. A tin of kaolin (the lid removed and contents well stirred).
3. A small pan in which to heat the kaolin (pan half-filled with water).
4. A spatula.
5. A piece of old linen cut and cornered.
6. A layer of gauze.

To apply—A tray with the following :

1. Two well-heated plates (between which to place the poultice).
2. A receiver with a piece of cotton-wool, a bandage and a safety-pin.

Whenever necessary—

A bottle of olive oil and a gallipot.
A gallipot with cotton-wool mops.
A receiver for soiled mops and previous poultice.

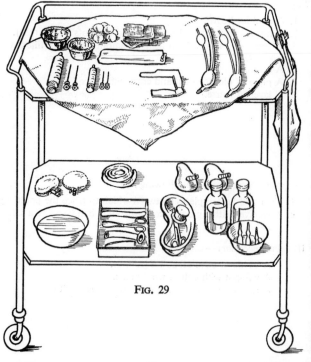

FIG. 29

FIG. 29
Trolley for electrotherapy (E.C.T.)

1. Sterile packet containing:
       One large disposable clinical sheet.
       Gauze swabs.
       Cotton-wool mops.
       Treatment drape.
       Two disposable gallipots.
2. 20 ml. syringe and needles (for intravenous anæsthesia).
3. 2 ml. syringe and needles (for giving muscle relaxant).
4. Laryngoscope.
5. Magill's cuffed endotracheal tubes.
Disposable paper bag taped to the side of the trolley to receive soiled swabs.
6. Electrodes (well padded with cotton-wool and gauze).
7. Bowl containing normal saline solution (to moisten electrode pads).
8. Small tray or receiver with:
       Tongue depressor.   Airway.
       Tongue forceps.   Mouth gag.
9. Receiver with adhesive tape and scissors.
10. Tourniquet.
11. Bottle of cetavlon (1 per cent.).
12. Bottle of skin hibitane.
13. Anæsthetic face masks.
14. Drugs to be used, *e.g.*, pentothal sodium or methohexital sodium (" brietal sodium "), scoline.

Other requisites:
       Electrotherapy machine.
       Cylinder with oxygen or oxygen and 5 per cent. carbon dioxide.
       Tray with syringes, needles and emergency drugs, *e.g.*, nikethamide or adrenalin hydrochloride.

(*N.B.*—All apparatus should be checked and tested before treatment is commenced.)

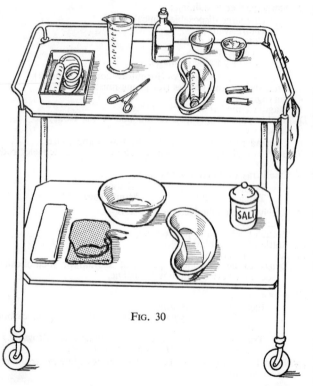

Fig. 30

FIG. 30

Trolley for glucose-interruption

(May be required when deep insulin coma is induced.)

1. Tray or large receiver with cylindrical funnel and an œsophageal tube No. 8 (sterile).
2. Clip or artery forceps for clamping the tube.
3. Graduated measure containing 600 ml. of 33 per cent. glucose.
4. Gallipot with gauze swabs.
5. Lubricant, *e.g.*, glycerine or liquid paraffin.
6. Gallipot for lubricant.
7. Receiver with 20-ml. syringe (for withdrawal of gastric juice).
8. Litmus paper (to test acidity of gastric juice before administration of the glucose).

If reaction is only slightly acid, 1 drachm of salt may be added to the glucose. This reduces the risk of chloride deficiency and may prevent vomiting.

9. Waterproof cape and a towel for protection of the patient.
10. Sickness basin.
11. Large receiver for tube and funnel after use.
12. Jar with salt.
13. Disposable paper bag taped to the side of the trolley to receive soiled swabs.

(*N.B.*—In some circumstances glucose-interruption may be by the intravenous method.)

NOTES

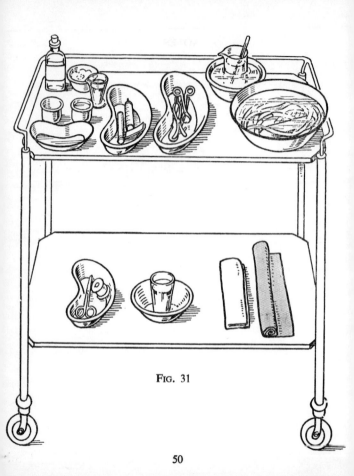

Fig. 31

FIG. 31

Trolley for intra-nasal or intra-oral œsophageal feeding

1. The apparatus, *e.g.*, a cylindrical glass funnel, a piece of rubber tubing, a glass connection and a fine rubber œsophageal tube (No. 20) sterilised and placed in a bowl of warm sterile water. (For the nasal method : a fine rubber œsophageal tube (No. 5 or 6) or, if for a child, a fine rubber catheter (No. 4 or 5).)
2. A measure containing the feed at the correct temperature, 100° F. (37·7° C.) standing in a bowl of warm water.
3. A food thermometer.
4. A large receiver with mouth gag, tongue forceps and a spatula.
5. A receiver with a 10 ml. record syringe and litmus paper.
6. A measure with warm sterile water.
7. A small bowl with cotton-wool mops.
8. A small bowl with boracic lotion.
9. A bottle of lubricant, *e.g.*, liquid paraffin or glycerine.
10. A gallipot for the lubricant.
11. A receiver for soiled swabs.

12. A tumbler with mouth wash and a sickness basin.
13. A receiver with scissors and adhesive strapping.
14. Polythene and disposable drape.

   (*Continuous feeding* by the drip method may be required.)

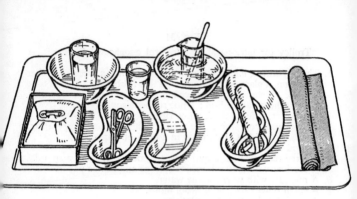

FIG. 32

Tray for a gastrostomy feed

1. A small tray with a packet containing sterile towels and dressings.
2. A receiver with two pairs of sterile dressing forceps.
3. A tumbler with mouth wash and a sickness basin.
4. A small measure with warm sterile water.
5. A receiver for soiled swabs.
6. A measure containing the feed, standing in a bowl of warm water to maintain it at the correct temperature, 100° F. (37·7° C.).
7. A food thermometer.
8. A large receiver with the sterile apparatus, *i.e.*, a cylindrical glass funnel, rubber tubing and a glass connection.
9. Polythene to protect clothing.

For a jejunostomy feed requirements are similar with the addition of an ointment to apply to skin.

(Continuous feeding may be given by drip method.)

NOTES

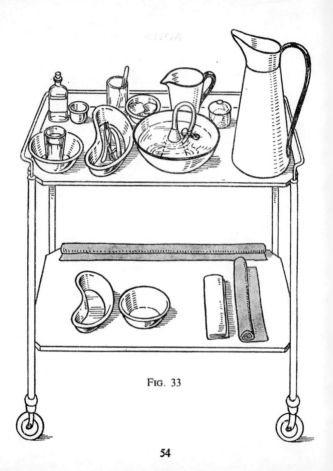

Fig. 33

FIG. 33

Trolley for a gastric lavage

1. A large basin with the sterile apparatus, *e.g.*, funnel, length of rubber tubing, glass connection, clamp and œsophageal tube (No. 16 to 20) in sterile water.
2. A bottle of liquid paraffin.
3. A gallipot for the lubricant.
4. A bowl of gauze swabs.
5. A receiver with a mouth gag and a tongue depressor.
6. A tumbler with a mouth wash and a bowl for the return.
7. A graduated jug.
8. A small bowl for the dentures.
9. A lotion thermometer.
10. A large jug with the solution, *e.g.*, 4 litres of solution of soda bicarbonate, temperature 100° F. (37·7° C.).

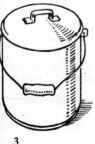

11. A receiver or disposal bag for soiled swabs.
12. A sickness basin.
13. Polythene and disposable drape.
14. A protection for the floor.
15. A bucket for the return wash.

3

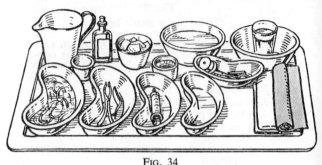

FIG. 34

Tray for intermittent gastric suction

1. A Ryle's tube and clip in warm sterile water.
2. Liquid paraffin and a gallipot.
3. A receiver with a 20 ml. syringe.
4. A graduated measure jug for the stomach contents.
5. A bowl with gauze swabs or linen squares.
6. A mouth wash and sickness basin.
7. A receiver or disposal bag for soiled swabs.
8. A denture jar.
9. A receiver with a mouth gag and spatula.
10. A bowl with water in which to rinse the syringe.
11. Receiver with adhesive tape, scissors and litmus paper.
12. Polythene and disposable drape.

(Continuous gastric suction may be carried out using Wangensteen's apparatus, electric suction apparatus, or " pipe line " suction.)

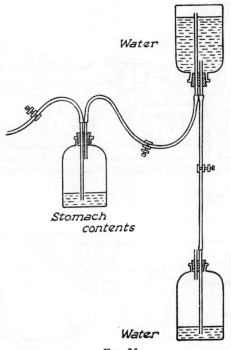

Water

Stomach contents

Water

Fig. 35

Wangensteen's apparatus for continuous gastric suction

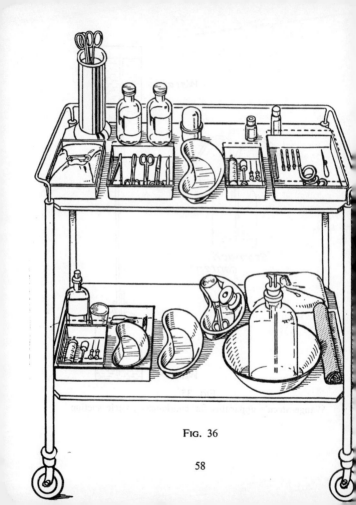

Fig. 36

Fig. 36

Trolley for the removal of fluid from the legs

(By acupuncture or by Southey's tubes.)

1. A jar with Cheatle's forceps.
2. A small tray with a packet of sterile towels and dressings.
3. A bottle of cetavlon, 1 per cent.
4. A bottle of methylated spirit.
5. Two sterile gallipots for the lotions.
6. Sterile hypodermic syringe and needles in syringe box or packet.
7. A bottle of local anæsthetic, *e.g.*, novocaine, 2 per cent.
8. A small tray with a pair of dissecting forceps, two pairs of dressing forceps, scissors, and scalpel or tenotomy knife (sterile and covered).
9. A receiver or bag for used instruments.
10. A sterile universal container for specimen of fluid.
11. A tray with several of the small Southey's cannulæ with pieces of fine rubber tubing attached. (For acupuncture: the tenotomy knife or a large cutting needle.)
12. A sterile packet with several large pads of gamgee tissue and gauze bandages (for acupuncture).
13. A basin with a sterile bottle for drainage of fluid from tubes.
14. Polythene to protect bed.
15. A receiver with scissors, adhesive strapping, and cotton thread.
16. A receiver or disposal bag for soiled dressings.
17. A stimulant tray with a bottle of brandy and a medicine glass, a hypodermic syringe and needles in box or packet, ampoules of adrenaline and coramine, a file, and a small receiver.

Before Puncture.—Fracture boards placed under the mattress and the skin cleaned and shaved.

(Omit Cheatle's forceps and modify as required when equipment is available from Central Sterile Supply Department.)

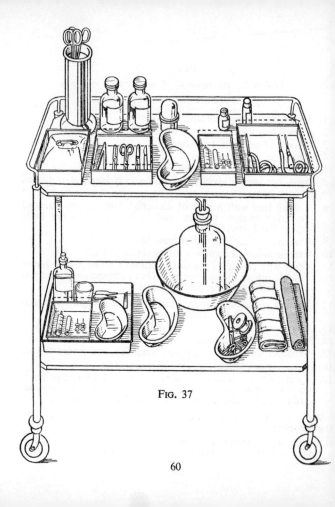

Fig. 37

Fig. 37
Trolley for paracentesis abdominis

1. A jar with Cheatle's forceps.
2. A small tray with a packet of sterile towels and dressings.
3. A bottle of cetavlon (1 per cent.).
4. A bottle of methylated spirit.
5. Two sterile gallipots.
6. A sterile hypodermic syringe and needles in syringe box or packet.
7. A bottle with local anæsthetic, *e.g.*, xylocaine (0·5 per cent.).
8. A small tray with a pair of dissecting forceps, two pairs of dressing forceps, scissors and a scalpel or tenotomy knife (sterile and covered).
9. A receiver or bag for soiled instruments.
10. A sterile universal container for specimen of fluid.
11. A tray with the apparatus, *e.g.*, a medium-sized trocar and cannula and a length of rubber tubing, or two Southey's tubes and pieces of fine rubber tubing (sterile and covered).

12. Polythene to protect bed.
13. A many-tailed abdominal binder.
14. A receiver with adhesive strapping, scissors and safety-pins.
15. A large basin and a Winchester bottle.
16. A receiver or disposal bag for soiled dressings.
17. A stimulant tray with a bottle of brandy and a medicine glass, sterile hypodermic syringe and needles in syringe box or packet, ampoules of adrenaline, coramine, a file and a small receiver.

(Omit Cheatle's forceps and modify as required when equipment is available from Central Sterile Supply Department.)

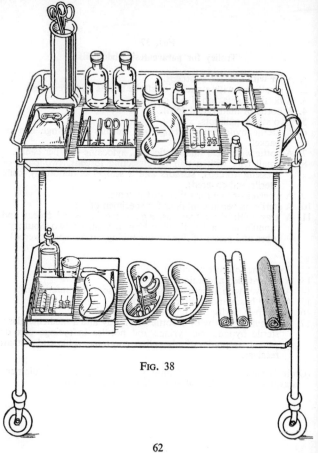

Fig. 38

Fig. 38

Trolley for aspiration of the pleural cavity

1. A jar with Cheatle's forceps.
2. A small tray with a packet of sterile towels and dressings.
3. A bottle of cetavlon (1 per cent.).
4. A bottle of methylated spirit.
5. Two sterile gallipots for the lotions.
6. Sterile hypodermic syringe and needles in syringe box or packet.
7. A bottle of local anæsthetic, *e.g.*, novocaine (2 per cent.).
8. A receiver or bag for used instruments.
9. A small tray with two pairs of dressing forceps, a pair of dissecting forceps and a pair of scissors (sterile and covered).
10. A sterile universal container for the specimen.
11. A measure for the fluid.
12. A tray or packet with sterile apparatus, *e.g.*, a 20 ml. syringe, two-way adaptor with small piece of rubber tubing attached to one arm, and suitable sized chest-exploring needles.

13. Polythene to protect bed.
14. A chest binder.
15. A receiver or disposal bag for soiled swabs.
16. A receiver with adhesive strapping, scissors and safety-pins.
17. A stimulant tray with a bottle of brandy and a medicine glass, a hypodermic syringe and needles in a box or packet, ampoules of adrenaline, coramine, a file and a small receiver.

(Omit Cheatle's forceps and modify as required when equipment is available from Central Sterile Supply Department.)

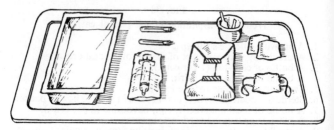

FIG. 39

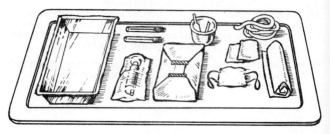

FIG. 40

64

Fig. 39

Tray for intramuscular injection

1. Sterile disposable foil tray.
2. Packet with sterile syringe.
3. Sterile needles of appropriate length and bore.
4. Sterile swab impregnated with skin antiseptic.
5. The drug to be given (this may be in an ampoule or rubber-capped bottle).
6. Ampoule file when necessary.
7. Face mask.
8. Sterile hand towel.

   (Check written prescription before administration.)

Fig. 40

Tray for intravenous injection

1. Sterile disposable foil tray.
2. Packet with sterile syringe.
3. Sterile intravenous needles (a cannula may be required for withdrawing a drug from ampoule).
4. Packet containing sterile towels.
5. Sterile swabs impregnated with a skin antiseptic or a bottle with skin antiseptic and packet of sterile cotton-wool mops.
6. Drug to be administered and ampoule file when necessary.
7. Some form of tourniquet, *e.g.*, a piece of rubber tubing or sphygmomanometer.
8. Protection for bed.
9. Face mask.

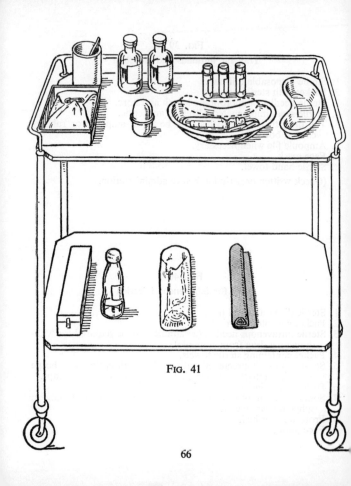

FIG. 41

Fig. 41

Trolley for venepuncture (for withdrawal of blood)

1. A small packet containing sterile towels and swabs.
2. A bottle of cetavlon (1 per cent.).
3. A bottle of methylated spirit.
4. Two sterile gallipots.
5. A large receiver or packet with the dry sterile intravenous needles and syringe (10 or 20 ml.).
6. A container with sterile dissecting forceps.
7. The required number of laboratory specimen jars.
8. A receiver or disposal bag for soiled swabs.

9. A sphygmomanometer.
10. A packet containing a blood-taking set if a large amount is to be withdrawn.
11. A bottle containing 100 ml. of 2·5 per cent. sodium citrate solution (anticoagulant).
12. A protection for the bed.
13. Face masks.

(A disposable blood " taking set " may be used.)

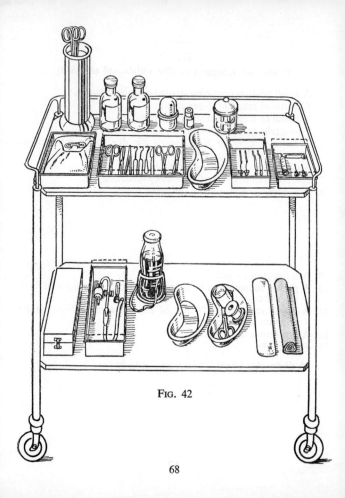

Fig. 42

Fig. 42
Trolley for venesection

1. A jar with Cheatle's forceps.
2. A small tray with a packet of sterile towels and dressings.
3. A bottle of cetavlon (1 per cent.).
4. A bottle of methylated spirit.
5. Two sterile gallipots for the lotions.
6. A bottle of local anæsthetic, *e.g.*, xylocaine (0·5 per cent.).
7. A covered tray with the required sterile instruments :
   - 2 Pairs of dressing forceps.
   - 1 Pair of dissecting forceps.
   - 2 Blunt hook retractors.
   - 1 Aneurysm needle.
   - 1 Scalpel.
   - 1 Pair of stitch scissors.
   - 2 Pairs of mosquito forceps.
8. Small packet or covered container with assorted sterile cannulæ, or a packet with an intracath.
9. A jar or foil pack with needles and suture material.
10. A syringe box or packet containing a 2 ml. syringe and hypodermic needles.
11. A receiver for soiled instruments.

12. A sphygmomanometer.
13. A bottle with blood or saline solution as required.
14. A transfusion " giving set " in covered box or packet.
15. A receiver or disposal bag for soiled dressings.
16. A receiver with a bandage, adhesive strapping and scissors.
17. A padded splint.
18. A protection for the bed.
19. Face masks.

(Omit Cheatle's forceps and modify as required when equipment is available from Central Sterile Supply Department.)

A disposable blood-pack unit may be available.

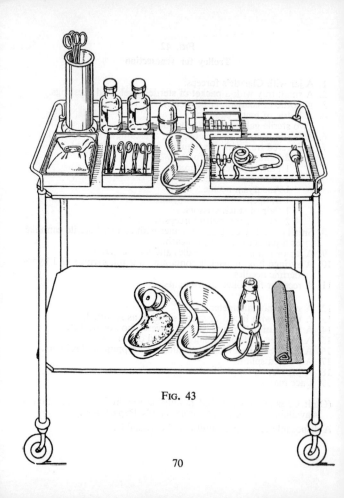

Fig. 43

Fig. 43
Trolley for subcutaneous infusion

1. A jar with Cheatle's forceps.
2. A small tray with a packet containing sterile towels, cotton-wool, gauze swabs and a pad of gamgee.
3. Bottles with the required lotions for cleaning and disinfecting the skin, *e.g.*, cetavlon (1 per cent.) and methylated spirit.
4. Sterile gallipots.
5. A bottle with local anæsthetic, *e.g.*, xylocaine (0·5 per cent.).
6. A sterile hypodermic syringe and needles in a box or packet.
7. A small receiver.
8. A covered tray with the following sterile instruments :
     2 Pairs of dressing forceps.
     1 Pair of dissecting forceps.
     1 Pair of dressing scissors.
9. A covered tray or autoclaved packet containing :
     Y-shaped glass connection.
     2 Short pieces of rubber tubing.
     2 Subcutaneous needles (bent and flat pointed).
     2 Clamps.
     Drip apparatus and tubing.

10. A bottle of warmed normal saline.
11. A protection for bed.
12. A receiver or disposal bag for soiled swabs.
13. A receiver with adhesive strapping and a large pad of warmed cotton-wool.
14. Face masks.

(Hyalase may be injected to promote absorption of fluid. A bed cradle should be at hand as required.)

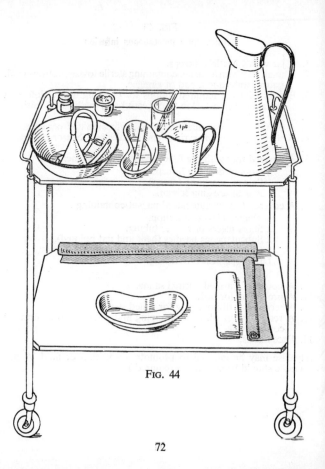

Fig. 44

Fig. 44

Trolley for a rectal lavage

1. A large bowl with the sterile apparatus, *e.g.*, a funnel, a length of rubber tubing, glass connection, rectal tube and clip.
2. A jar of petroleum jelly and wooden spatula.
3. A bowl with cotton-wool mops.
4. A receiver or disposal bag for soiled mops.
5. A lotion thermometer.
6. A measuring jug (600 ml. capacity).
7. A large jug with the wash-out lotion, *e.g.*, 3-4 litres of normal saline solution, temperature 105° F. (40·5° C.).

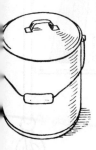

8. A protection for the floor.
9. A receiver for soiled rectal tube.
10. A disposable drape.
11. A protection for the bed.
12. A bucket for the return wash.

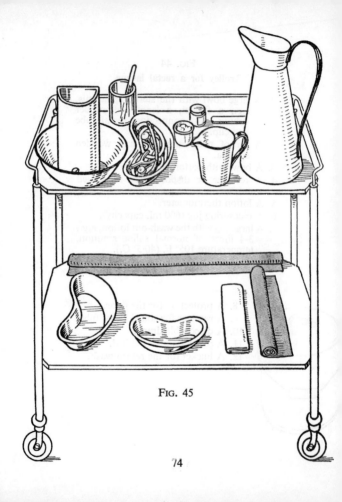

Fig. 45

FIG. 45

Trolley for colonic lavage

1. A large bowl with a sterile graduated irrigation can (a funnel may be used).
2. A large receiver with the remainder of the sterile apparatus, *e.g.*, two pieces of rubber tubing, a Y-shaped glass connection, two clamps and a rectal tube.
3. A jar of petroleum jelly and a wooden spatula.
4. A small bowl with cotton-wool mops.
5. A lotion thermometer.
6. A measuring jug (600 ml. capacity).
7. A large jug with the wash-out lotion, *e.g.*, 3-4 litres of normal saline solution, temperature 105° F. (40·5° C.).

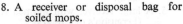

8. A receiver or disposal bag for soiled mops.
9. A receiver for soiled rectal tube.
10. A protection for the floor.
11. A disposable drape and protection for the bed.
12. A bucket for the return wash.

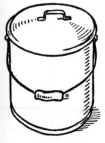

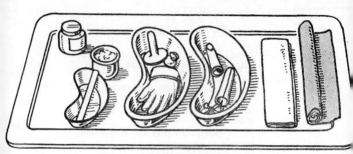

FIG. 46

Tray for rectal examination

1. A jar of petroleum jelly and wooden spatula.
2. A bowl of cotton-wool mops.
3. A receiver or disposal bag for soiled mops.
4. A receiver with rubber gloves and a small bag of French chalk (a caped finger stall may be used).
5. A large receiver with warmed rectal speculum (Ferguson's or Cusco's).
6. A disposable drape.
7. A protection for the bed.

(A hand lamp may be required.)

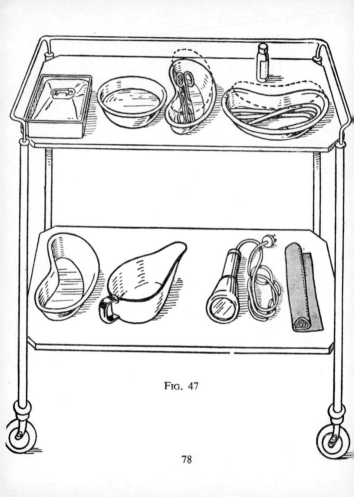

FIG. 47

Fig. 47

Trolley for the catheterisation of the urinary bladder of a female patient

1. A small tray with a dressing packet containing sterile towels, cotton-wool and gauze swabs.
2. A bowl of warm antiseptic lotion for swabbing the vulva.
3. A receiver or suitable container with three pairs of sterile dressing forceps.
4. A covered receiver or catheter tray with three sterile catheters (No. 8) or three disposable catheters.
5. A sterile jar if laboratory specimen is required.

6. A receiver or disposal bag for soiled swabs and catheters.
7. A suitable-sized graduated receptacle for urine.
8. A hand lamp.
9. A protection for the bed.
10. Face mask.

(Additional requirements if self-retaining catheter is to be introduced.)

Sterile self-retaining urethral catheter and introducer.
Sterile water for cuff and 20-ml. syringe for introduction of water to cuff.
Sterile drainage tube or spigot.
Adhesive tape.

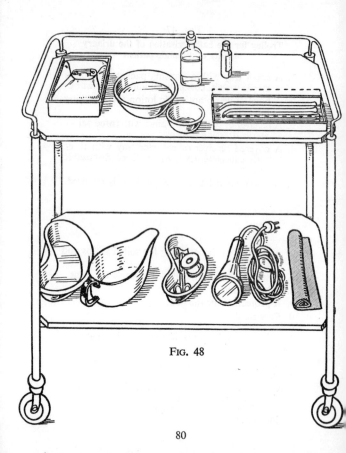

FIG. 48

FIG. 48

**Trolley for the catheterisation of the urinary bladder of a
male patient**

1. A small tray with a dressing packet containing sterile towels,
   cotton-wool and gauze swabs.
2. A bowl of antiseptic lotion for swabbing the external parts.
3. A bottle with sterile lubricant, or a tube of K.Y. jelly.
4. A sterile gallipot for lubricant if required.
5. A sterile covered catheter tray with an assortment of sterile
   catheters as required.
6. A sterile jar if laboratory specimen is required.

7. A large receiver or disposal bag for soiled swabs and catheters.
8. A suitable-sized graduated receptable for urine.
9. A receiver with scissors, adhesive strapping and, if the catheter
   is to be tied in position, a roll of tape and a spigot.
10. A hand lamp.
11. A protection for the bed.
12. Face mask.

(When self-retaining catheter is to be introduced, see additional
   requirements as listed with Fig. 47.)

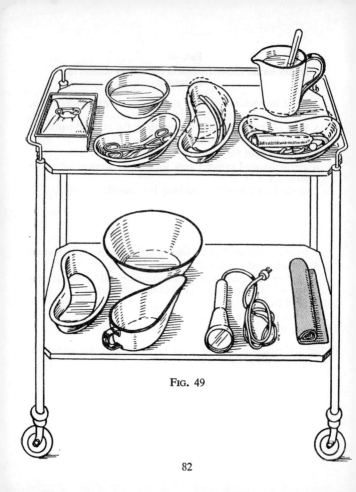

FIG. 49

FIG. 49

Trolley for bladder lavage in female patient

1. A small tray with a packet containing sterile towels, cotton-wool and gauze swabs.
2. A bowl of warm antiseptic lotion for swabbing the external parts.
3. A receiver or suitable container with three pairs of sterile dressing forceps.
4. Two or three sterile rubber catheters (No. 8) in a covered receiver or catheter tray (or pack with disposable catheters).
5. A measure with 1,100 ml. of sterile irrigation lotion, *e.g.*, normal saline, temperature 100° F. (37·7° C.).
6. Lotion thermometer.
7. A large receiver or packet with the sterile apparatus, *i.e.*, cylindrical funnel, tubing, connection and clamp (bladder syringe for the suction method).

8. A receiver or disposal bag for soiled swabs and catheters.
9. A suitable sized receptacle for the urine.
10. A large bowl or bucket for the return wash.
11. A hand lamp.
12. A protection for the bed.
13. Face mask.

Bladder lavage in the male patient.—Requirements as for catheterisation plus funnel and tubing as above or a bladder syringe.

Continuous bladder irrigation may be carried out using tidal-drainage apparatus as illustrated in Fig. 50.

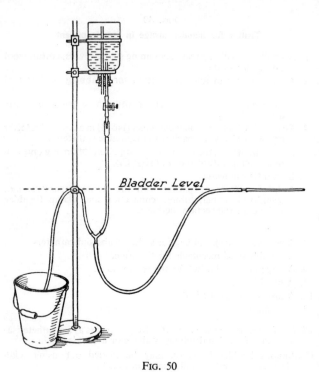

Bladder Level

FIG. 50

Tidal drainage

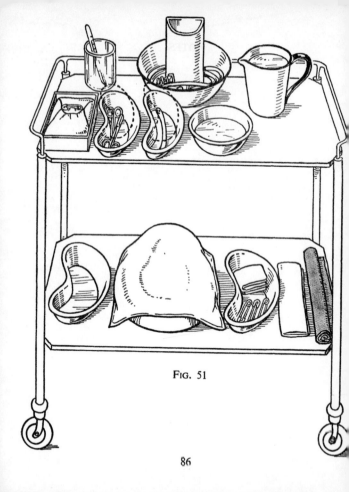

FIG. 51

Fig. 51

Trolley for vaginal douche

1. A tray with a small packet of sterile dressings, *e.g.*, gauze and cotton-wool swabs, dressing towels, and perineal pads as required.
2. A receiver or suitable container with three pairs of dressing forceps.
3. A packet or covered receiver with sterile douche nozzle.
4. A bowl with warm antiseptic lotion for swabbing the vulva.
5. The douche can, a length of rubber tubing and a clamp, sterilised and in a large bowl.
6. A measure jug containing two to four pints of the sterile solution at the required temperature (varies, depending on purpose for which douche is given).
7. A lotion thermometer.

8. A receiver or disposal bag for soiled swabs.
9. A bed pan or douche pan and cover.
10. A receiver with T-bandage and safety-pins if necessary.
11. A protection for the bed.

Face mask, gown and cap should be worn by the nurse.

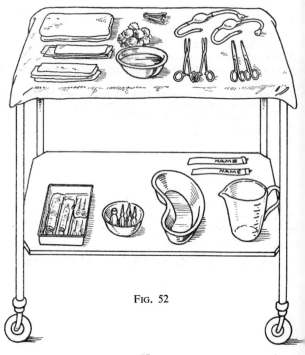

FIG. 52

Fig. 52
Trolley for normal delivery

1. Sterile packet containing:
        Baby wraps.
        Drapes.
        Perineal pads.
        Cotton-wool mops.
2. Bowl containing swabbing lotion.
3. 2 pairs of 7 in. Spencer Wells forceps.
4. 2 pairs of straight Mayo scissors.
5. 1 disposable umbilical clamp.
6. 2 Mucus extractors.

7. Small tray or receiver with one 20 ml. and one 2 ml. syringe and needles.
8. Drugs, *e.g.*:
        Duncaine (0·5 per cent. solution).
        Syntometrine (1 ml.).
        Ergometrine (0·5 mg.).
        Intravenous ergometrine (0·125 mg. (2 ampoules)).

9. Large receiver.
10. Graduated jug (1 litre).
11. 2 identification bands (clip seal).

Other requisites—
        2 hand lotion basins.
        Sterile packs with hand towel, gown and gloves.
        Disposal bag for discarded swabs.
        Prepared, heated basket or cot.

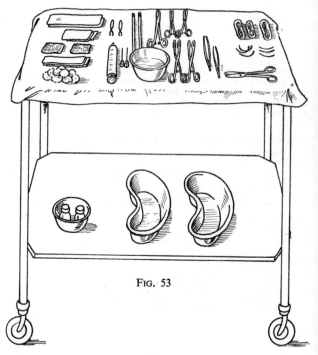

Fig. 53

FIG. 53

Trolley for repair of perineum

1. Sterile packet containing:
>> Perineal pads.
>> Stitch pads.
>> Gauze swabs.
>> Drapes.
>> Cotton-wool mops.

2. One 20 ml. syringe and needles.
3. Bowl containing swabbing lotion.
4. 2 pairs of swab-holding forceps.
5. 2 catheters (No. 7).
6. 2 towel clips.
7. 1 needle holder.
8. 2 pairs of small artery forceps.
9. 2 pairs of dissecting forceps (one toothed, one non-toothed).
10. 1 pair of stitch scissors.
11. Needles (round-bodied No. 2 and cutting Nos. 2 and 3).
12. Catgut (No. 1 and 2). Black silk (No. 1 and 2).

13. Local anæsthetic, *e.g.*, duncaine (0·5 per cent. solution).
14. 2 large receivers.

Other requisites—
>> Hand lotion basin.
>> Sterile packs with hand towel, gown and gloves.
>> Disposal bag for discarded swabs.

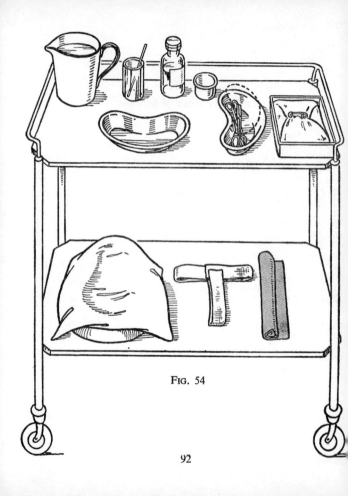

Fig. 54

FIG. 54

Trolley for jug douching and perineal care

1. A measuring jug with 1,000 ml. of warm antiseptic solution, *e.g.*, aqueous hibitane 1 in 2,000.

2. A lotion thermometer.

3. A suitable container or covered receiver with three pairs of sterile dressing forceps.

4. A tray with a small packet containing sterile towels, gauze and cotton-wool swabs and a vulval pad.

5. A bottle of antiseptic as required, *e.g.*, skin hibitane (an antibiotic powder may be required).

6. A sterile gallipot.

7. A receiver or disposal bag for soiled swabs, etc.

8. A sterile douche pan and a cover.

9. A T-bandage.

10. A protection for the bed.

(A lamp should be at hand when necessary and a chest blanket.)

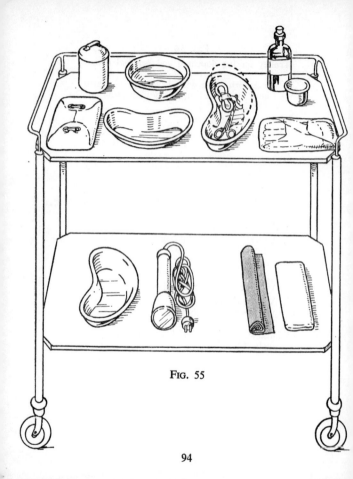

F<small>IG</small>. 55

94

Fig. 55

Trolley for insertion of pessaries

1. A packet of sterile towels.
2. A jar or packet with sterile swabs.
3. A bowl of warm antiseptic lotion, *e.g.*, aqueous hibitane 1 in 2,000.
4. A receiver or disposal bag for soiled swabs.
5. A covered receiver with, *e.g.*, a rubber-covered watch spring pessary, a length of tape and a pair of artery forceps or a special introducer. (Other types of pessaries which may be used—vulcanite ring, Hodge's or ring and stem.)
6. A bottle with a sterile lubricant, *e.g.*, liquid paraffin and a gallipot (hibitane cream may be used).
7. A packet with a pair of sterile rubber gloves.

8. A protection for the bed.
9. A lamp.
10. A receiver for discarded gloves when not of disposable type.

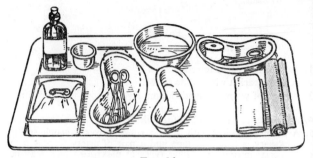

FIG. 56
Tray for the insertion of a tampon

1. A small tray with packet containing sterile towel, vulval pad, tampon and cotton-wool mops.
2. A bowl of warm antiseptic lotion, *e.g.*, aqueous hibitane 1 in 2,000.
3. A receiver or disposal bag for soiled swabs, etc.
4. A covered receiver with two pairs of dressing forceps and a pair of swab-holding forceps.
5. A bottle containing the prescribed solution (in which to soak tampon).
6. A sterile gallipot.
7. A receiver with adhesive strapping and a pair of scissors.
8. A protection for the bed.

(Ensure a good light—using a bell lamp if necessary.)

NOTES

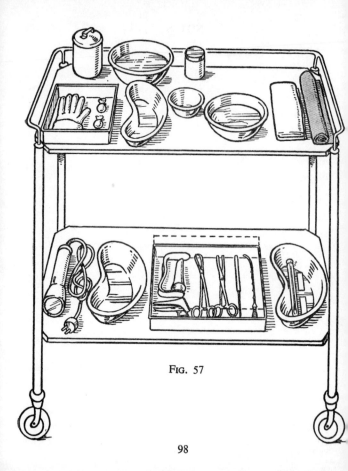

FIG. 57

98

Fig. 57

Trolley for vaginal examination

Upper shelf (if for digital examination only)—

1. Small tray with packet containing sterile rubber gloves and dusting powder.
2. A jar or packet of cotton-wool mops.
3. A bowl of warm antiseptic lotion, *e.g.*, aqueous hibitane 1 in 2,000.
4. A jar with lubricant, *e.g.*, obstetric cream, and a gallipot.
5. A receiver or disposal bag for soiled swabs.
6. A bowl with antiseptic lotion in which to place used gloves when not of disposable type.
7. A protection for the bed.

Lower shelf (when visual examination is necessary)—

1. A covered tray with :

    Vaginal specula, *e.g.*, Cusco's, Sim's and Ferguson's.
    Single-toothed vulsellum forceps.
    Swab-holding forceps.
    A Playfair's probe.
    A uterine sound.

2. A receiver for soiled instruments.
3. A receiver with cervical swab and slides if specimen is required.
4. A lamp.

A suitable fixative should be available to cover slides as required.

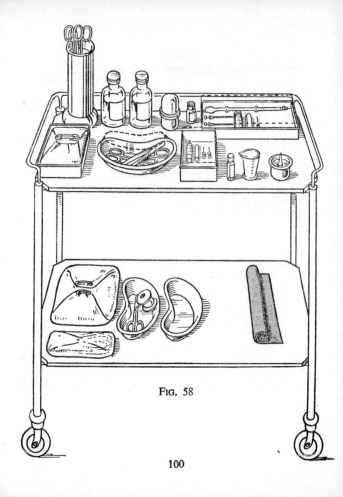

FIG. 58

FIG. 58

Trolley for lumbar puncture

1. A jar with Cheatle's forceps.
2. A small tray with a packet containing sterile towels and dressings.
3. A bottle of cetavlon (1 per cent.).
4. A bottle of methylated spirit.
5. Two sterile gallipots.
6. A covered receiver or suitable container with three pairs of sterile dressing forceps.
7. Hypodermic syringe and needles in syringe box or packet.
8. A bottle with local anæsthetic, *e.g.*, novocaine (2 per cent.) or xylocaine (0·5 per cent.).
9. Two lumbar puncture needles, a spinal manometer, 10 or 20 ml. syringe and cannula; these may be autoclaved in a packet or a special covered tray. A tenotomy knife may also be required.
10. A sterile specimen bottle.
11. A small glass measure for the fluid.
12. When a drug is being introduced intrathecally, the ampoule may be standing in a bowl of warm water to heat it to body temperature.

13. A receiver with adhesive strapping and scissors.
14. A receiver or disposal bag for soiled swabs.
15. A protection for the bed.
16. Packets containing sterile gowns, masks and gloves.
17. A stimulant should be at hand.

(Alternative method of preparing trolley when for spinal anæsthesia is shown in Fig. 61.)

For cisternal puncture or ventricular puncture—Requirements are similar, but the appropriate needle is substituted for the lumbar puncture needle.

(Omit Cheatle's forceps and make necessary modification when equipment is available from Central Sterile Supply Department.)

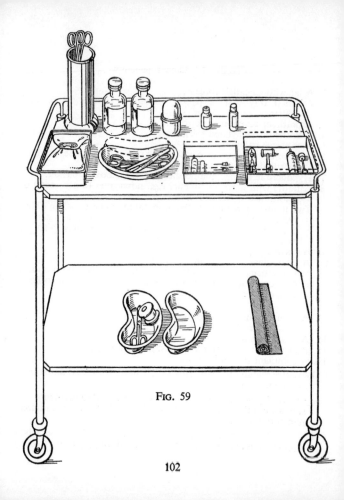

Fig. 59

FIG. 59

Trolley for sternal puncture

1. A jar with Cheatle's forceps.
2. A small tray with a packet containing sterile towels and dressings.
3. A bottle of cetavlon (1 per cent.).
4. A bottle of methylated spirit.
5. Two sterile gallipots for the lotions.
6. A syringe box or packet with sterile hypodermic syringe and needles.
7. A bottle of local anæsthetic, *e.g.*. xylocaine (0·5 per cent.).
8. A covered receiver or suitable container with three pairs of sterile dressing forceps.
9. A small tray or packet with the autoclaved apparatus—A sternal puncture needle in a glass tube, small mallet and a 10 ml. syringe.
10. One or two sterile heparinised tubes for specimen or, when necessary, glass slides.

11. A receiver with adhesive strapping and scissors.
12. A receiver or disposal bag for soiled swabs.
13. A protection for the bed.
14. A stimulant should be at hand.

(Omit Cheatle's forceps and make necessary modification when equipment is available from Central Sterile Supply Department.)

Face masks and gowns should be worn.

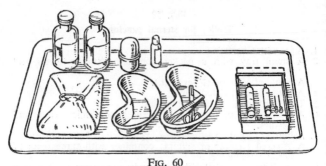

Fig. 60

Tray for local anæsthetic by injection

1. Small packet containing sterile towel and swabs.
2. A bottle with cetavlon (1 per cent.).
3. A bottle of methylated spirit.
4. Two sterile gallipots.
5. Bottle containing the local anæsthetic, *e.g.*, xylocaine (0·5 per cent.).
6. Packet or box with 5 and 2 ml. dry sterile syringes and assorted suitable sized needles.
7. A receiver or suitable container with three pairs of sterile dressing forceps.
8. A receiver or disposal bag for soiled swabs.

(Local anæsthesia may also be produced using, *e.g.*, a spray or drops.)

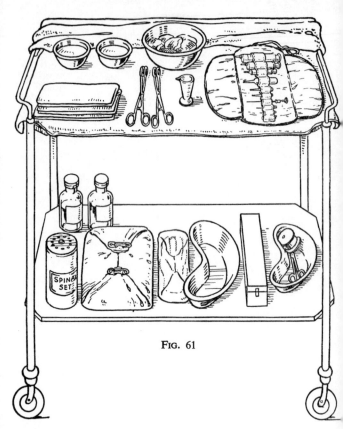

FIG. 61

FIG. 61
Trolley for spinal anæsthesia

Sterile towel on trolley—
1. A gallipot with hibitane and cetavlon.
2. A gallipot with skin hibitane.
3. A bowl with sterile gauze swabs.
4. Two swab-holding forceps.
5. Sterile towels.
6. A small measure or gallipot for cerebrospinal fluid.
7. A spinal bundle containing :
    - (*a*) 1 20 ml. syringe.
    - (*b*) 1 10 ml. syringe.
    - (*c*) 1 2 ml. syringe.
    - (*d*) 1 ampoule of heavy spinal nupercaine.
    - (*e*) 1 ampoule of light spinal nupercaine.
    - (*f*) 1 ampoule of 0·5 per cent. xylocaine.
    - (*g*) 2 lumbar puncture needles.
    - (*h*) 2 large wide-bore needles for emptying ampoules.
    - (*i*) 2 hypodermic needles.
    - (*j*) An ampoule file.

    (This bundle is autoclaved at 20 lb. pressure at a temperature of 260° F. (126·6° C.) for twenty minutes.)

    (*All ampoules must be discarded and renewed before resterilising as the drug must be autoclaved once only.*)

8. Bottles with lotions for skin.
9. Small drum from which spinal set is removed.
10. Gowns, caps, masks and gloves for anæsthetists.
11. Receiver for discarded equipment.
12. Sphygmomanometer.
13. Adhesive strapping and scissors.
14. Disposal bag for soiled dressings.

(A sterile spinal manometer should be at hand. Trolley covered with a sterile towel.)

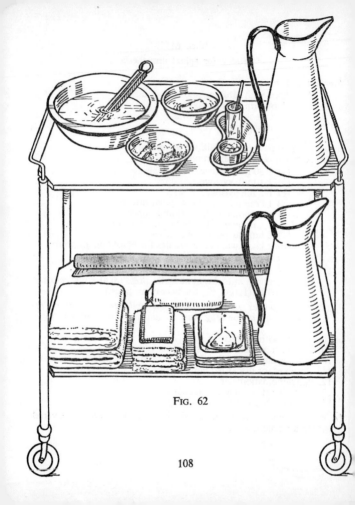

Fig. 62

FIG. 62

Trolley for tepid sponging

1. A basin of water, temperature 70° to 80° F. (21·1° to 26·6° C.).
2. A bath thermometer.
3. A bowl with six sponges or washing flannels.
4. A bowl with iced water and a compress for the forehead.
5. A receiver with a clinical thermometer and cotton-wool mops.
6. Two large jugs with water.

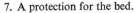

7. A protection for the bed.
8. Two bathing sheets.
9. Two bath towels and a face towel.
10. Clean nightdress and bed linen as required.
11. A hot water bottle in a cover.
12. A bucket for soiled water.
13. A receptacle for soiled linen.

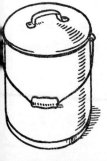

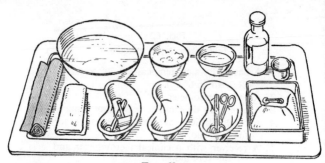

FIG. 63

Tray for pre-operative skin preparation

1. A bowl of hot water.
2. A bowl with cotton-wool and gauze swabs.
3. A receiver with a razor and a pair of scissors.
4. A small bowl with warm ether soap.
5. A receiver or disposal bag for soiled swabs.
6. A protection for the bed.
7. A disposable drape.

When a skin disinfectant and sterile dressing is to be applied add :—

      (*a*) A bottle with the ordered disinfectant, *e.g.*, hibitane.
      (*b*) A gallipot for the lotion.
      (*c*) A receiver or suitable container with set of dressing
          forceps.
      (*d*) A small packet containing the necessary sterile dressings
          and towels.

NOTES

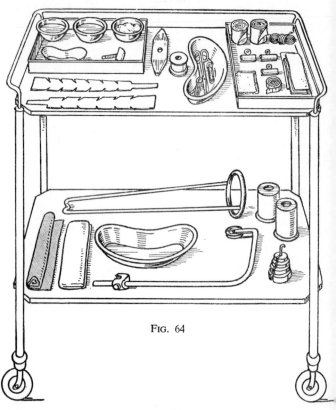

FIG. 64

112

Fig. 64

Trolley for application of skin traction

1. A small tray with requisites for shaving the limb if necessary: small bowls containing warm water, ether soap and cotton-wool mops, a razor and a small receiver.
2. Prepared strips of orthopædic adhesive strapping.
3. A wooden spreader and a roll of adhesive strapping.
4. A receiver with scissors and safety-pins.
5. A tray with domette and calico bandages, flannel slings and paper clips, strong cord, a tape measure, and chiropodist felt or other suitable padding material.

6. A protection for the bed.
7. Weights, pulleys and extension pole as required.
8. Bed blocks.
9. A splint, *e.g.*, Thomas's splint.
10. A receiver or disposal bag for discarded materials.

(Fracture boards are placed underneath the mattress as required, a large bed cradle and bed elevator should be at hand.)

A Ventfoam traction kit may be used as a temporary measure in application of skin traction or when patient's skin is not suitable for use of adhesive strapping.

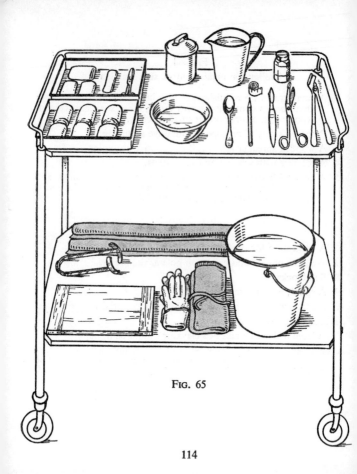

F<small>IG</small>. 65

114

FIG. 65
Trolley for the application of plaster of Paris

1. A small tray with the necessary plaster bandages.
2. A small tray with stockinet of suitable width, cotton-wool bandages, orthopædic felt or sorbo padding and a pair of dressing scissors.
3. A tin with dry plaster and a plaster spoon.
4. A bowl for plaster cream.
5. A jug of warm water.
6. A tape measure and skin pencil.
7. A tin of glove powder.
8. Plaster shears (if old plaster is being removed), plaster scissors and knife.

9. A bucket or large deep bowl with tepid water in which to soak the plaster bandages.
10. A protection for the floor.
11. A protection for the bed as required.
12. Mackintosh apron and rubber gloves.
13. A suitable sized board if slabs require to be made.
14. Any appliances which may require to be incorporated in the plaster, *e.g.*, walking iron, heel or Cramer wire, etc.

(Fracture boards under the mattress and large bed cradle at hand when necessary.)

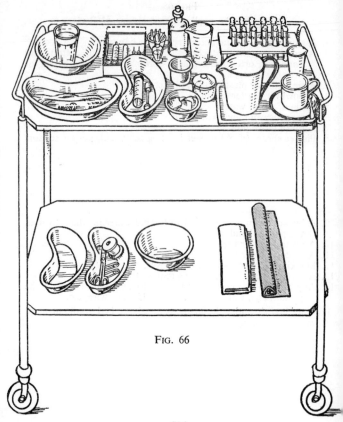

FIG. 66

116

Fig. 66
Trolley for fractional test meal

1. A receiver with a sterile Ryle's tube and clip immersed in warm sterile water.
2. A receiver with a 10 or 20 ml. syringe.
3. A tumbler with a mouth-wash and a bowl for the return.
4. A bottle of liquid paraffin.
5. A gallipot for the lubricant.
6. A bowl of gauze swabs.
7. A small bowl for the dentures.
8. A measure for the fasting gastric juice.
9. A rack with twelve numbered test tubes.
10. A measure for the residual juice.
11. A hypodermic syringe and needles in box or packet.
12. An ampoule of histamine and file.
13. A bottle of Töpfer's solution.
14. A small tray with the test meal, *e.g.*, a jug with gruel and a saucer and teaspoon.

15. A receiver or disposal bag for soiled swabs.
16. A receiver with adhesive strapping, safety-pins and scissors.
17. A sickness basin.
18. A protection for the bed.

Various types of test meals may be ordered. Those in common use include :

Histamine (0·5 mg.) given subcutaneously.

Histamine (0·4 mg.) per 10 kg. of body weight augmented by giving 4 ml. of antistin intramuscularly thirty minutes beforehand.

Alcohol, *e.g.*, 50 ml. of 7 per cent. alcohol.

NOTES

NOTES

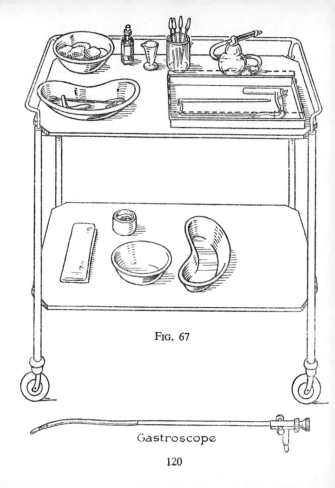

Fig. 67

Gastroscope

Fig. 67

Trolley for œsophagoscopy

1. A bowl of gauze swabs.
2. A bottle with the local anæsthetic, *e.g.*, cocaine (10 per cent.).
3. A suitable measure for the anæsthetic.
4. A jar with dressed wooden probes.
5. De Vilbiss spray.
6. A receiver with angled tongue depressor and grasping forceps.
7. A tray with the apparatus :
>   Œsophageal speculum.
>   Œsophagoscope.
>   Detachable suction tube.

8. Sickness basin.
9. Denture jar.
10. Receiver or disposal bag for soiled swabs.
11. A disposable drape.
12. Biopsy specimen bottle when required.

(*N.B.*—Patient premedicated. Local anæsthesia may be supplemented by intravenous pentothal. Suction apparatus and œsophageal tubes to hand.)

For gastroscopy—Substitute gastroscope for œsophagoscope.

(The required anæsthesia may be produced by giving local anæsthetic lozenges to suck.)

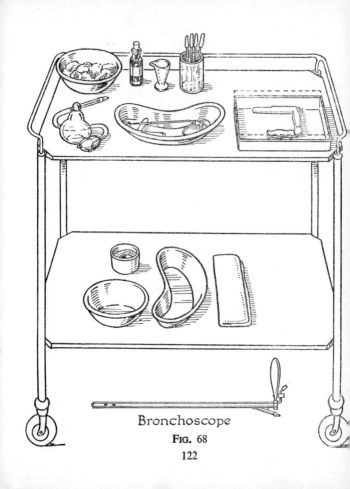

Bronchoscope

FIG. 68

FIG. 68

Trolley for direct laryngoscopy

1. A bowl of gauze swabs.
2. A jar with dressed wooden probes.
3. A bottle with the local anæsthetic, *e.g.*, cocaine (10 per cent.).
4. A suitable measure for the anæsthetic.
5. De Vilbiss spray.
6. A small tray with laryngoscope(s).
7. A receiver with angled tongue depressor and grasping forceps.

8. Sickness basin.
9. Denture jar.
10. A receiver or disposal bag for soiled swabs.
11. A disposable drape.

(*N.B.*—Patient premedicated. Several sizes of laryngoscope available. Extra electric bulbs at hand. Suction apparatus in readiness.)

(It may be necessary to have tracheotomy instruments also in readiness.)

For bronchoscopy—Requirements are similar with the addition of a bronchoscope.

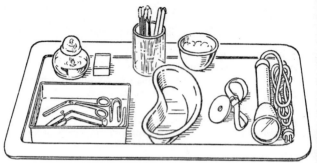

FIG. 69

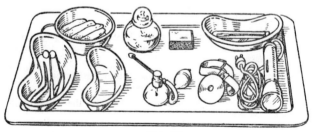

FIG. 70

124

Fig. 69

Tray for the examination of the nose and nasopharynx

1. A small tray with a nasal speculum, angular dressing forceps, post-nasal mirrors and a tongue depressor.
2. A spirit lamp and matches.
3. A receiver or jar containing wooden probes which have been dressed with cotton-wool, and several wooden spatulæ.
4. A bowl of cotton-wool swabs.
5. A receiver for used instruments.
6. A forehead mirror.
7. A lamp.
8. A disposal bag for soiled swabs.

Fig. 70

Tray for examination of the throat and larynx

1. A receiver with tongue depressor and laryngeal mirrors.
2. A bowl with tongue cloths, *e.g.*, folded pieces of gauze or linen.
3. A spirit lamp and matches.
4. A receiver for used instruments.
5. A forehead mirror and lamp.
6. A sterile throat swab in a receiver.
7. A De Vilbiss spray and local anæsthetic when necessary.
8. A disposal bag for soiled gauze, etc.

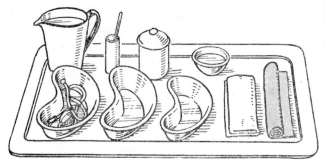

FIG. 71

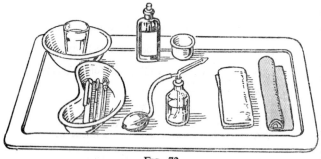

FIG. 72

Fig. 71

Tray for irrigation of the nose

1. A jug containing 500 to 1,000 ml. lotion, *e.g.*, normal saline or soda bicarbonate, 1 : 160 solution, temperature 100° F. (37·7° C.).
2. A lotion thermometer.
3. The sterile apparatus which may be a rubber syphon douche or a rubber ball syringe.
4. A jar with cotton-wool swabs.
5. A small bowl of boracic lotion for swabbing the nostrils.
6. A receiver or disposal bag for soiled swabs.
7. A receiver for the return wash.
8. A protection for bed and patient.

Fig. 72

Tray for irrigation and painting of the mouth and throat

1. A glass of gargling fluid and a bowl for the return.
2. A bottle containing throat paint, *e.g.*, Mandl's paint, and a gallipot.
3. A receiver with a torch spatula, camel-hair brush and a throat swab if necessary. (Swab taken before any treatment is given.)
4. A throat spray with the solution ordered.
5. A protection for bed and patient.

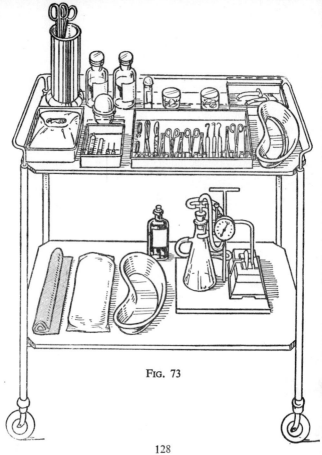

FIG. 73

128

Fig. 73

Trolley for tracheotomy

1. A jar with Cheatle's forceps.
2. A tray with a packet containing sterile towels, gauze swabs and key-hole dressings cut ready for round the tracheostomy tube.
3. The required lotions for cleaning and disinfecting the skin, *e.g.*, cetavlon (1 per cent.) and methylated spirit.
4. Sterile gallipots for lotions.
5. Local anæsthetic, *e.g.*, xylocaine (0·5 per cent.).
6. Sterile hypodermic syringe and needles in a box or packet.
7. A covered instrument tray with the following sterile articles :—
   - 2 Towel clips.
   - 1 Scalpel.
   - Sponge-holding forceps.
   - 6 Pairs of small artery forceps.
   - 1 Single hook retractor (blunt).
   - 1 Double hook retractor (blunt).
   - 1 Single hook retractor (sharp).
   - 1 Pair of tracheal dilators (Bowlby's).
   - 1 Pair of pointed scissors.
   - 1 Needle holder.
8. Tracheostomy tube complete, *i.e.*, outer tube with tapes, inner tube and pilot.
9. A container with curved round-bodied and cutting needles.
10. A jar with suture material, *e.g.*, catgut and silk.
11. A receiver with rubber catheter for suction.
12. Suction apparatus and antiseptic for use with same, *e.g.*, solution of Milton (5 per cent.).
13. A receiver for used instruments.
14. A small sandbag in cover.
15. A protection for the bed.
16. A disposal bag for soiled swabs.

(Sterile gowns, masks and gloves will be provided for the surgeon. A bronchoscope should be to hand, also a cylinder of oxygen, and carbon dioxide (7 per cent.). Omit Cheatle's forceps and modify requirements when equipment is available from Central Sterile Supply Department.)

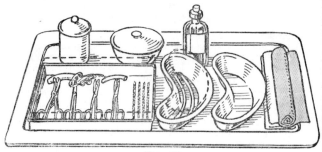

FIG. 74

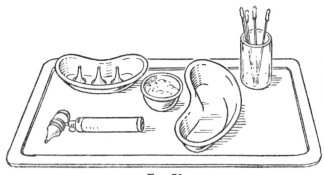

FIG. 75

Fig. 74

Tray for after-care of a tracheotomy

1. A covered jar or bowl with the necessary sterile dressings, *e.g.*, gauze swabs and cut dressings for insertion between the skin and tube.
2. A bowl with a saturated solution of sodium bicarbonate.
3. A covered tray with the following sterile articles :
    An exact duplicate of the tracheostomy tube complete with tapes and pilot in position.
    Tracheal dilators.
    Pointed scissors.
    2 Pairs of dressing forceps.
    Several pipe cleaners.
4. Covered bowl or receiver with two soft rubber catheters.
5. A receiver or disposal bag for soiled material.
6. A bottle with antiseptic solution for use with suction apparatus, *e.g.*, solution of Milton (5 per cent.).
7. A protection for the bed.

(Oxygen and carbon dioxide (7 per cent.) should be at hand with the suction apparatus.)

Fig. 75

Tray for examination of the ear

1. An electric auriscope.
2. A receiver with assorted aural specula.
3. A jar or receiver with wooden probes dressed with cotton-wool.
4. A bowl with cotton-wool swabs.
5. A receiver or disposal bag for soiled cotton-wool.
6. A receiver for used specula.

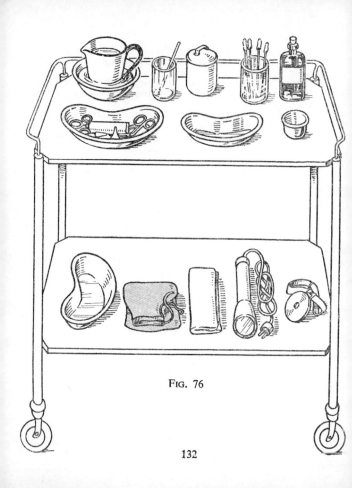

FIG. 76

Fig. 76

Trolley for syringing and swabbing the ear

1. A jug of lotion, *e.g.*, normal saline or sodium bicarbonate 1 : 160, standing in a bowl of warm water to maintain it at the correct temperature, 100° F. (37·7° C.).
2. A lotion thermometer.
3. A jar with cotton-wool swabs.
4. A receiver or disposal bag for soiled swabs.
5. A large receiver containing an aural syringe, rubber aural tip, aural speculum and angled forceps. (A Higginson's bulb syringe and eustachian catheter may also be used.)
6. A jar or receiver with wooden probes dressed with cotton-wool.
7. A bottle with the prescribed solution and a gallipot when necessary.

8. A large receiver for the return wash.
9. A waterproof shoulder cape.
10. A disposable drape.
11. A lamp.
12. A forehead mirror.

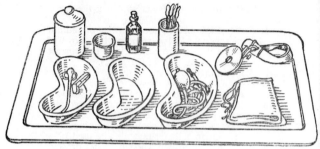

Fig. 77

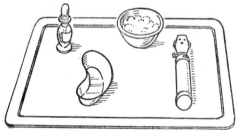

Fig. 78

FIG. 77

Tray for inflation of the middle ear

1. A jar with cotton-wool swabs.
2. A receiver with eustachian catheter and nasal speculum.
3. A bottle with cocaine (10 per cent.) and gallipot.
4. A jar with dressed probes.
5. A Politzer bag and auscultation tube.
6. A receiver or disposal bag for soiled dressings.
7. A shoulder cape.
8. A forehead mirror.

FIG. 78

Tray for examination of the eye

1. Eye-drop bottle containing a solution of atropine or homatropine as ordered.
2. Bowl of cotton-wool swabs.
3. Receiver or disposal bag for soiled swabs.
4. Electrically illuminated ophthalmoscope.

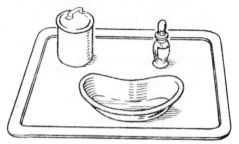

FIG. 79

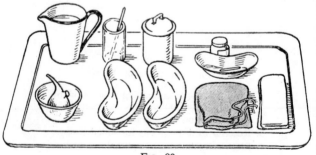

FIG. 80

FIG. 79

Tray for instillation of eye drops

1. A jar or packet with superfine cotton-wool swabs.
2. A receiver or disposal bag for soiled swabs.
3. Eye drops in a bottle with pipette attached to stopper.

N.B.—Careful check to be made of drops used. Patients may
   have own individual drop bottles or single dose opulets may
   be available.

FIG. 80

Tray for irrigation of the eye and the application of an ointment

1. A jug containing 300 ml. of sterile lotion, *e.g.*, normal saline,
   temperature, 100° F. (37·7° C.).
2. A lotion thermometer.
3. A sterile undine irrigator in a sterile bowl.
4. A jar or packet with sterile superfine cotton-wool swabs.
5. A receiver for soiled swabs.
6. A receiver for the return wash.
7. A waterproof shoulder cape.
8. A disposable drape.

When an ointment is to be applied—Add a jar with the ointment and
   a small receiver with a glass eye rod. (Single dose opulets may
   be available.)

When irrigating an eye in acute infections, e.g., *gonorrhœal
   ophthalmia*—Add a pair of rubber gloves and goggles (to be
   worn by the nurse).

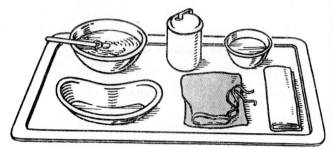

Fig. 81

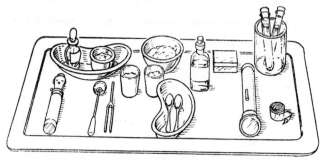

Fig. 82

Fig. 81

Tray for swabbing and spoon bathing of eye

1. A bowl of hot water.
2. A wooden spoon padded with cotton-wool.
3. A jar or packet of cotton-wool swabs.
4. A small bowl of lotion for swabbing, *e.g.*, boracic lotion or normal saline.
5. A receiver or disposal bag for soiled swabs.
6. A waterproof shoulder cape.
7. A small towel.

Fig. 82

Tray for neurological examination

1. A receiver with small bowl of cotton-wool mops and a bottle containing eye drops as ordered, *e.g.*, homatropine.
2. An ophthalmoscope.
3. A patella hammer.
4. A tuning fork.
5. A bowl with wisps of cotton-wool.
6. Small jars containing salt and sugar.
7. Teaspoons in a receiver.
8. A bottle containing, *e.g.*, oil of cloves.
9. A small box with pins.
10. A tape measure.
11. A pocket torch.
12. Test tubes containing hot and cold water.

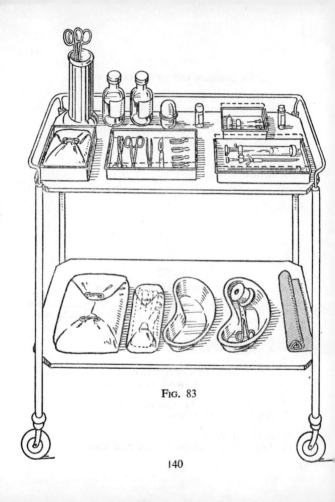

FIG. 83

FIG. 83

Trolley for liver biopsy

1. A jar with Cheatle's forceps.
2. A small tray with a packet containing sterile towels and cotton-wool and gauze swabs.
3. The required number of sterile gallipots and bottles with skin disinfectants, *e.g.*, methylated spirit, cetavlon and thio-mersalate, or hibitane and cetavlon, and skin hibitane.
4. Bottle with local anæsthetic, *e.g.*, procaine (1 per cent.) or xylocaine (0·5 per cent.).
5. Syringe box or packet with sterile hypodermic syringe and needles.
6. Covered instrument tray with :
   - 2 Pairs of dressing forceps.
   - 1 Pair of dissecting forceps.
   - 1 Scalpel.
   - 4 Towel clips.

7. Packet or tray with the sterile apparatus :
   - Liver puncture syringe fitted with trocar, cannula and guard (length of trocar approx. 5 in. ; bore, 1·5 mm.).
   - Probe for removing piece of liver tissue from cannula.

8. Laboratory specimen jar containing a fixative, *e.g.*, formal saline.

9. Packet containing sterile gown and mask.
10. Pair of surgeon's sterile gloves.
11. Receiver or disposal bag for soiled swabs.
12. Receiver with adhesive tape and scissors.
13. A protection for the bed.

(This procedure may be carried out using a 20 ml. syringe and suitable sized trocar and cannula.)

(*N.B.*—Before biopsy the blood group and prothrombin time should have been determined. A pint of blood should be ready if there is the possibility of bleeding.)

(Omit Cheatle's forceps and modify requirements when equipment is available from Central Sterile Supply Department.)

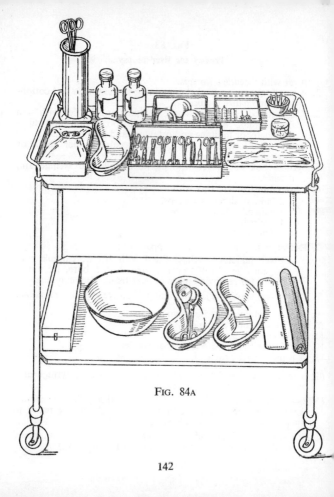

FIG. 84A

Number 1 trolley for cardiac catheterisation

1. A jar with Cheatle's forceps.
2. Small tray with packet containing sterile towels and swabs.
3. Bottles with the required lotions for skin, *e.g.*, methylated spirit, and thiomersalate.
4. Small tray with sterile gallipots inverted on it.
5. A 2 ml. syringe and needles in box or packet.
6. Small receptacle containing xylocaine (0·5 per cent.), procaine (1 per cent.), adrenaline (1 : 1,000) and an ampoule file.
7. Linen or plastic packet containing autoclaved cardiac catheter(s).
8. Covered tray with the required sterile instruments :

       Towel clips.
       Scalpel and blades.
       2 Pairs of artery forceps.
       2 Pairs of mosquito forceps.
       1 Pair of dissecting forceps.
       1 Aneurysm needle.
       1 Pair of Mayo's scissors.
       1 Pair of stitch scissors.

9. A small receiver or foil tray for resting instruments in.
10. Receptacle with nylon or silkworm gut and skin needles.

11. Sphygmomanometer.
12. Bowl for catheter.
13. Receiver with adhesive tape and scissors.
14. Receiver or disposal bag for discarded material.
15. Padded arm splint.
16. A protection for the bed.

(Omit Cheatle's forceps and modify requirements when the equipment is available from Central Sterile Supply Department.)

(For remaining requirements see Fig. 84b.)

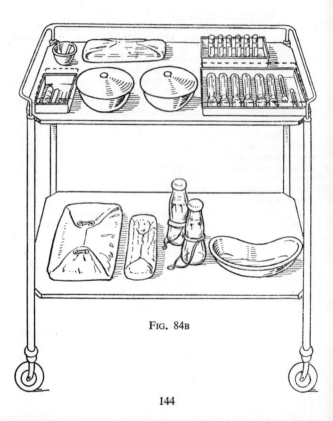

Fig. 84b

Number 2 trolley for cardiac catheterisation

1. Packet with autoclaved drip set and fittings.
2. Ampoule of heparin, hypodermic syringe and needles.
3. Two covered lotion bowls.
4. Tray containing six 20 ml. autoclaved syringes and two wide bore needles.
5. Small tray with six sterile tubes containing liquid paraffin for the specimens of blood.

6. Large receiver for discarded syringes.
7. The required number of bottles containing heparinised saline or normal saline.
8. Packets containing sterile gowns, caps and gloves.
   (Drip stand and manometer in metal tube should be at hand.)

NOTES

146

NOTES

NOTES

STERILISATION

The Medical Research Council Memorandum 15 placed great stress on the need for central syringe services and the importance of reliable sterilisation procedures. It stated that "all medical students and nurses should be taught safe methods of sterilisation, and they must know the risks that attend careless and imperfect technique."

In the absence of a central supply service it becomes the nurse's responsibility to ensure that all equipment used for aseptic procedures has been rendered sterile.

Autoclaving or the use of hot air ovens are the methods of choice when complete bacteriological sterility is required.

Although the need for some measure of standardisation has been recognised and its early establishment very desirable, there still remains a wide range of methods in common use.

In view of the fact that much research is at present in progress and pending further recommendations from the Medical Research Council, all methods of sterilisation should be kept under constant review. No attempt could be made here to enumerate all methods or select any one as being ideal, generally accepted, practice. The following suggestions, however, may prove helpful in the preparation of equipment for tray and trolley setting.

Some general rules to be observed.

Preliminary cleansing of all articles must be thorough if adequate results are to be obtained from any method of sterilisation (ultrasonic washers are sometimes available).

All sterile articles must be handled with sterile forceps or clean sterile-gloved hands (non-touch technique).

In all measures taken to prevent the spread of infection thorough washing and drying of the hands must not be overlooked. When preparing to carry out or assist with aseptic procedures, *e.g.*, ward dressings, the hands should be washed thoroughly in warm soapy water, rinsed (preferably under running water) and dried carefully.

A clean towel is all that is necessary for drying unless sterile gloves have to be worn, when a sterile towel should be used. Prolonged *scrubbing*, which removes protective substances, etc., from the skin and is injurious to the tissues, should be avoided. No surgical work should be carried out with hands which are dripping with water or a disinfectant solution as this could be a possible source of infection.

Before packing needles, syringes and instruments, etc., they must be carefully examined to ensure that needles are not blocked and have sharp points, that syringes all have matching barrels and pistons, that instruments are undamaged and in working order.

Adequate wrapping should be provided to prevent breakages and the points of needles and cutting edges of sharp instruments must be protected.

Outer cotton or linen wrappings should be at least double thickness and must be kept clean and free from holes.

Dressing packets, etc., should not be too large, should be loosely packed, securely wrapped and clearly marked. When safety-pins are used to secure packets, only the outer layer of material should be pierced in order to avoid contamination of the contents on removal of the pin.

Drums or cardboard boxes must never be packed too tightly and great care should be taken to ensure that no part is defective.

All sterile packages and drums should be labelled with the date of sterilisation and if not opened will require to be resterilised at the end of two to four weeks, giving consideration to the type of material forming the outer covering. All sterile packets and boxes should be stored in a warm, dust-free cupboard and be subjected to the minimum of handling while in storage.

Ensure that rubber gloves have been repaired, powdered and paired as required.

Water sterilisers should be emptied completely at least once per day, and be thoroughly cleaned before refilling.

Absolute cleanliness of tray or trolley to be used must be ensured.

Methods commonly used.

Autoclaving (steam pressure sterilising).—Steam under pressure, at the required temperature, is delivered to the chamber containing articles to be sterilised. These chambers must not be too tightly packed and adequate steam penetration of all articles must be ensured.

Temperature, pressure and time of exposure will vary with the materials to be sterilised. Timing should never commence until the desired temperature has been reached within the chamber. Drying time is important.

Spore envelopes or reliable control tubes should be placed in the autoclave regularly in order to check the efficiency of the apparatus and method. These should be put in the centre of packages and drums.

Articles which may be sterilised by this method include :

> Metal instruments, bowls, basins, trays and jugs, etc.
> Dressing materials, gowns and linen, etc.
> Glassware, *e.g.*, syringes, jars and flasks, etc.
> Suture materials, *e.g.*, silk, nylon and wire.

These are usually subjected to a temperature of 250° to 260° F. (121·1° to 126·6° C.), 15 to 20 lb. extra pressure for twenty minutes.

Rubber goods such as catheters, tubing and gloves, etc., are usually subjected to a temperature of 240° to 250° F. (115·5° to 121·1° C.), 10 to 15 lb. extra pressure for ten to fifteen minutes.

A high pressure instrument autoclave may be available. This employs extra pressure of 30 to 32 lb. per square inch, giving a temperature of approximately 134° C. The actual sterilising time is two to three minutes and the whole procedure need only occupy five to seven minutes.

Hot Air Ovens.—There are two types : electric convection ovens and infra-red radiant heat. The high temperature reached in these ovens is unsuitable for dressing materials and other articles which would be destroyed by such long exposure to strong dry heat. Their use is therefore more limited than that of the autoclave.

Articles which may be sterilised by this method include :

> All glass syringes, needles, laboratory test tubes and flasks, etc.
> Soft and liquid paraffins.
> Glove powder.
> Sharp instruments and those not suitable for autoclaving.

These are usually subjected to a temperature of 160° C. for one hour.

Boiling water sterilisers.—These should be of suitable size to allow complete immersion of all articles to be sterilised. A perforated tray may be used to facilitate removal of equipment. Always ensure that light rubber goods are not just floating on the surface.

The use of a thermometer attached to the steriliser is the most accurate method of determining when the water is boiling, as it may appear to boil on the surface before it has reached a temperature of 212° F. (100° C.). When no thermometer is attached do not commence timing until the water appears to boil vigorously. No articles should be added to the contents of the steriliser while the boiling period of others is being timed.

The addition of sodium bicarbonate to form a 2 per cent. solution increases the lethal effect of boiling and prevents corrosion of metal instruments.

This method is not recommended as suitable for sterilising syringes or needles. (These should be treated in the autoclave or hot air oven whenever practicable.)

Articles which may be sterilised by this method include :

Metal articles such as bowls, basins, jugs and instruments, etc.
Glassware such as funnels, measures, bottles and jars, etc.
Strands of suture materials, *e.g.*, nylon.
Rubber goods such as catheters, tubing and teats, etc.

Although bacteriological tests have shown that a two-minute boiling period is sufficient to ensure destruction of all pathogenic bacteria except those that produce resistant spores, to allow a margin of safety five minutes is considered a standard time.

Articles made of gum elastic or neoplex and nylon are usually boiled for two to three minutes.

Chemicals.

These are used much less for the purpose of sterilising equipment than any of the other methods mentioned. They should only be used in an emergency or when the required equipment cannot be sterilised by heat. It must be borne in mind that their effectiveness is considerably reduced in the presence of organic material (blood, pus

152

and oil, etc.), therefore all articles must be very carefully cleaned before immersion.

There is an extremely wide range of chemical agents available, and when choosing one the following should be well understood :

Its antibacterial properties.

The strength in which it is effective.

The minimum contact period required to render articles sterile.

The serious risks involved when chemicals are used at dilutions, or under circumstances which cause them to be ineffective.

Whether or not they are injurious to the tissues.

The possibility of adverse effects on equipment which might result from prolonged exposure.

Chemicals in common use include :

Cetavlon (1 per cent.) is suitable for preliminary cleansing of equipment and for skin disinfection. It may also be combined with hibitane to enhance its antiseptic action. It is considered to be one of the most suitable antiseptic detergents available to-day.

Hibitane at suitable dilutions has proved effective for use in :

Emergency disinfection of instruments, e.g., 0·5 per cent. solution in 70 per cent. isopropyl. Time of exposure, five to ten minutes. This allows a good margin of safety, as bacteriological tests have shown that a two-minute period will destroy pathogenic organisms (does not destroy spores).

Sterilisation of cystoscopes and other non-boilable endoscopy apparatus, e.g., a 1 : 5,000 aqueous solution. Time of immersion, thirty minutes.

Storage of sterilised sutures, e.g., 1 : 2,000 solution in water or spirit.

Formalin is useful for the sterilisation of gum-elastic goods and also delicate instruments which cannot be subjected to heat. It may be used as a 1 per cent. solution or as formalin vapour. In the case of the latter a special container is used, into a compartment of which are placed formalin tablets, approximately one tablet per 3 cub. in. of space in the container. The instruments must be clean and dry before being placed in the box. After exposure for twelve to twenty-four hours they are rinsed in sterile water before use. If an electric formalin steriliser is available, the vapour is formed much more rapidly and articles may be sterilised in ten to fifteen minutes.

Dettol is an extremely useful disinfecting agent and has the advantage of being non-toxic and non-irritant. It is frequently used in the following dilutions :

1 : 20, *e.g.*, wound disinfection.

1 : 40, in obstetrics, for hands and general disinfection of wards and theatres, etc.

1 : 160, *e.g.*, vaginal douching and swabbing.

5 per cent. solution in spirit, *e.g.*, for rapid disinfection of instruments in an emergency (two minutes' immersion).

1 per cent. solution in spirit, *e.g.*, rubber goods can be immersed in this for long periods without suffering any adverse effects.

Dettol obstetric cream, a non-greasy ointment, extremely useful as an antiseptic in midwifery.

Specialised sterilisation techniques include the use of:

1. **Ethylene Oxide.** This requires special chambers where a high vacuum can be produced and a concentration of ethylene oxide in carbon dioxide introduced at a carefully controlled pressure which is above atmospheric pressure. This method of sterilisation is extremely effective against all microbial life including spores. It is useful for materials which are heat sensitive, *e.g.* plastics and equipment used in endoscopy. Apparatus such as heart lung machines may be sterilised by this method.

2. **Gamma Radiation.** Equipment necessary for this method of sterilisation remains extremely costly, but gamma rays from a Cobalt 60 source are being quite widely used for sterilising much of the disposable materials supplied to hospitals to-day, *e.g.* syringes, needles, catheters, tubing, blood taking and giving sets, etc.

INDEX

Printed in Great Britain at THE DARIEN PRESS, *Edinburgh*

Fasting Calcium

20mls. blood in 4 plain tubes.